Proven Systems For

Profitable Dental Hygiene

Proven Systems For

Profitable Dental Hygiene

John A. Wilde, D.D.S.

GP Publications
Batesville, AR 72503

First printing 2001

ISBN 0-9709932-1-8

DEDICATION

This book is dedicated to the superb dentists, hygienists and team members who strive diligently in the endless and seemingly un-winnable war against the active bacterial infection called gum disease. Each is a true warrior, never discouraged, no matter how many stinging defeats he or she may suffer, willing every day to rise again and fight the good fight.

And to my family, wife Joann, children Rachel, Megan, Heather, John Jr. and darling grandson, little Hunter John. They are the loves of my life, my inspiration, and the power and reason behind all I do.

ACKNOWLEDGEMENT

A portion of the proceeds from the purchase of each copy of *Profitable Dental Hygiene* will be donated to Scholarships for Life, a non-profit organization dedicated to helping find a cure for cancer.

If you are interested in obtaining more information about Scholarships for Life or would like to contribute to the ongoing work, please contact:

Scholarships for Life*
525 Lawrence Street
Batesville, AR 72501
870-698-2655

* Scholarships for Life is a special fund of The Mary Anne Evans & Lynda Cesarski Foundation for Cancer Research which has been registered with the U.S. Internal Revenue Service and the State of Arkansas as a 501 (c)(3) charitable organization.

CONTENTS

FOREWORD

by Dr. Woody Oakes

Dr. John Wilde has studied the "numbers" of private practice dentistry better than anyone I know. In this highly detailed book, he'll share with you the secrets of making your hygiene department three to four times more profitable.

You see, John has developed a **system** (over the past 15 years) that produces amazing results! A system that shows "average" dentists and hygienists how to take hygiene from a "loss leader" to a low-overhead "profit center."

In fact, using John's system, **one** hygienist and an assistant can add $98,000 to $100,240/year **NET** income to your practice. (That number is actually more than some practices' total NET income...practices that produce $500 K!)

Now there are a lot of people on the lecture circuit talking about how they used to do it, hope to do it, or dreamed about doing it. Sadly, many dentists buy into their advice without questioning its validity.

Conversely, everything John talks about in his book he's actually accomplished. He can document every statement and every dollar amount to the penny...he's got nothing to hide. And his focus is always on NET income, not on those other numbers that are as meaningless as hot air.

I know of no other seminar, audio tape, video tape or book that equals what John shares in this incredible book.

INTRODUCTION...

I hope you'll forgive me....

My goal--the intent of this book--is to significantly improve the lives of its readers. I feel achieving anything less is not worthy of your time, or mine. (Modest aspirations simply don't excite me.)

If the information I share, concerning the development of an ideal hygiene department as well as various and sundry other related topics, is to have such a profound impact, you must believe me. To trust my words, you must come to know me...to discover who I am and in what I most deeply believe. With this purpose in mind, I intend to reveal assorted facts concerning my personal and professional history throughout this text.

I wish to warn you that I'm an extremely candid person. I won't bore or mislead you with impotent generalities--this is good, that is better. What you'll receive from me are documented results of what I've accomplished in my life and dental practice. I begin our relationship by asking for your pardon and compassion, as I fear that some will feel such self-revelation to be bragging. I'm a humble and rather shy person, and to be considered guilty of self-serving arrogance would be extremely painful for me, but that's a risk I'm compelled to take.

Please understand that these revelations are simply describing myself and my practice as accurately and honestly as possible, to facilitate your ability to completely understand, evaluate and, if you so choose, implement my ideas. I'm aware that many dental practices have been vastly more successful than my little country office, their results dwarfing my greatest efforts and accomplishments. I consider myself an average or below average dentist skill-wise, and that's on my good days. (Of which there seem to be damn few!!)

But, as we say in Iowa, "even a blind pig finds an occasional acorn." During my 53 years extant, 28 of those invested as a practicing dentist, I've discovered a couple of modest things that have turned out rather well. I'd like to discuss some of these revelations with you. One of these successes involved developing a hygiene department that offered excellent patient care, while being extraordinarily profitable. (It is not coincidence that the most outstanding facet of my practice exists within a system in which I'm not directly involved in offering care. And I have enough to do, so I am very grateful for this fact.)

Before dealing directly with hygiene, let me attempt to introduce myself in a manner I believe will enhance the impact of my message. I apologize to the faithful readers of my other four dental books who have already suffered through some portions of my life story. (Hi Mom!)

I was born December 14, 1946--one of the oldest baby boomers--in the town of Lansing, Iowa. (Population 1,000...more if you count cows and other livestock.) I am the oldest of five siblings. Dad worked most of his career in a button factory. Mom returned to teaching high school when she felt her last child, my baby brother Jerry, was old enough to thrive without her, about the time I left for college.

I entered the University of Iowa in 1964. My parents had helped me fill out financial aid forms the previous year, and were pleased to discover that, with Dad working a second job and Mom working part time, they had an annual income in excess of $5,000--for the first time ever!

The good portion of that information was that I qualified for financial aid, I'd guess with quite a bit of room to spare. (The bad part--raising a family of seven on $5,000 annual income, even considering inflation adjustment--should be self-evident. I have no idea how my folks managed, but we were never in debt, and living for many years sans money creates in one a visceral and unforgettable awareness of its powers that has served me well.)

I don't know how this came to be, but, despite our family's fiscal reality, I can't recall a time when I didn't know I was going to college (brother Jim is an M.D., brother Jerry a Ph.D., so I guess they always knew too). It seems I also always knew I'd have to pay my own bills for higher education.

Despite this arguably innate awareness, I loafed around until age 8, when I accepted a job as a paper boy. I still remember holding up a hand full of coins for my customers to select their change. I'm sure I'd never had a dollar bill of my own, and hadn't yet learned how to make change. For three years, on all of the 365 days in each, I arose before school, or early mornings of days off, in weather ranging from blistering heat to sub-zero temperatures, to deliver my papers.

I abandoned this exciting and lucrative career track in the publishing industry at age 11, to begin working 70 hours a week, during summers, at the boat marina located directly across from our home. I worked nine-hour days Monday through Friday, then about 14 hours on Saturdays and Sundays, not getting a break for breakfast (I opened at 6 A.M.), lunch or dinner. My first year's salary was paid at a rate of 35 cents an hour. (My darn boss must have paid what my work was worth! I should have joined a union.)

After five years at the marina, jobs in factories, hardware stores, power plants, a gas station, hayfields, sawmills, then later as a campus policeman, lab research assistant and prison guard preceded my dental school graduation. The point was I worked--usually on difficult jobs, performed under tough conditions, for modest remuneration--but hey, at least the hours were long! And as I worked--beginning with coins from my paper route, stored in a glass fruit jar secured on a top kitchen shelf--I always saved money.

I wouldn't want any of my children to be forced to put forth quite this level of effort, but there are a lot worse things for a kid to learn than how to work hard. (Come to think of it, this regimen might be pretty good "basic training" for dentists! I can almost promise that a single day spent working with 200-pound-plus railroad ties in a hot, noisy, dirty, dangerous sawmill will put dentistry in a different perspective...and eliminate a lot of the whining.)

It damn near takes a moving van to relocate my lovely daughters to college. Despite my years of labor, I entered the University of Iowa with all my worldly possessions easily fitting into a single suitcase borrowed from my Aunt Dodie.

I recall late-night dormitory conversations, where my friends and I shared pizza and tentative visions of our futures. My secret desire was to some day make $10,000 a year. (I'm sure this goal was much too outrageous for me ever to state aloud.) Making twice my family's income was as wild a dream as I could envision. (Today $10,000 barely covers a week of family vacation to Utah skiing, or to the Virgin Islands.) I also hoped to one day be able to go into a restaurant for a meal and not even care what the food I ordered cost. (That dream came true--except for maybe a couple of places I've dined in Chicago--but now I have to worry about calories!)

I graduated from the University of Iowa College of Dentistry in 1972. I'd been responsible for 100 percent of my expenses for eight years, plus being married for the final three years to my lovely bride, Jo. We (actually she) had a child--John Jr.--a year and a half before I graduated. While blessed with a son, neither of us was blessed with any type of medical insurance.

When we wed, Jo's parents generously offered to buy an Iowa City home for us to inhabit free of all costs. After our graduation, they would keep the property for rental income, so it would be a great deal for us, and good for them. I said NO! Despite the fact that, after five years of college, I had no money, I also refused to let them pay for Jo's last year of education as a medical technologist. (Explanation for these decisions: I was nuts! I was raised poor but proud. Despite what you might have heard, that isn't really a very effective combination. Testosterone can be as deadly a drug as crack!)

Despite Jo's additional year of education expenses, childbirth and child-raising costs, and, as a family man, actually having to buy some (used) furniture, I owed $4,700 in total debt when I graduated and entered the United States Army Dental Corps. I was also intimately familiar with the feelings one acquires after several days without sleep.

In case I've been too subtle (which ain't real likely!), let me stomp squarely on the primary point I wish to make. Somehow, my parents' forced frugality had allowed me to understand innately that **debt is mortgaging one's future to pay for the present.** I sacrificed greatly during my educational career, but I did manage to achieve my educational goal, while keeping my future out of hock.

After two restful years of military duty in scenic Fort Lewis, Washington--my first experience with 40-hour weeks since age 11--Jo, John Jr., baby Heather and I started a practice from scratch on August 17, 1974, in that world-renowned hotbed of fine dentistry--Keokuk, Iowa.

During most of my two years of military service, I was actively involved in our search for an ideal practice location. I wrote, called, visited local dental offices and supply houses, and studied everything I could find (little existed then) concerning how to begin a private practice. We spent almost all our leave time (military paid vacation) touring Iowa (the state I love, and the only one in which I was licensed in those pre-regional board days), evaluating potential practice opportunities.

We lived in Keokuk for two months while the office I had envisioned and designed was under construction. During this interval, I interviewed and hired two staff members, and visited every dentist, physician, pharmacist and real estate agent in the area. There existed such an acute shortage of dentists in the Keokuk area that patients called our apartment to schedule appointments well before our practice opened, and months before we were listed in the phone book. Our hard work and due diligence paid immediate dividends, as our practice was fully booked from the first day we opened the office doors.

I had completely paid off all debt on my two-operatory office by March, 1975--less than eight months after we first opened the doors. This feat was accomplished due to a booming practice, while the four of us lived shoehorned into an modest upstairs two-bedroom apartment, spending very little money. My urge to consume was reduced by my working six extremely full days a week. I was delighted to rest on the Sabbath.

We moved into a new country home in May of 1975, within ten months of first opening our office doors. Despite my reluctance to borrow--even for a home--our office being completely paid for, plus a steady and increasing stream of revenue pouring from the practice, made the house obviously affordable. The new home was much nicer than the metal huts we'd inhabited in college, or even our military base housing! We'd paid our entire home debt off by 1978--after four years in private practice--at which time our family was completely debt-free, and started saving in earnest. I've never borrowed money since our house loan was repaid.

I still live in that same home, still with that same wife...although a child moves out occasionally. This trend may indicate I lack imagination, but sticking with my first wife, and our first home, have been two significant keys to my having achieved financial freedom relatively early. (I contend that it would be helpful if, when faced with major life decisions, every dentist would consider these pivotal choices in the light of how many more years I will be forced to work, if I choose to.....)

Here's a major point I don't want anyone to fail to grasp: most of my writing, and all of my life, have centered around a core theme of thoughtful, productive work, and unwavering fiscal responsibility. (Cheap seems a harsh word.)

There exists a clear pattern, in many facets of my life (that I'm sadly old enough to discern), revealing consistent efforts directed toward continual improvement. Discovering ways to do things better excites me! I'm a growth junkie! That paradigm of working toward constant progress defined my office, and resulted in the systems that have produced--along with a plethora of other innovative and lucrative behaviors--our ultra-successful hygiene department.

Let me again caution the unwary reader, we're preparing to openly discuss **net figures, and personal growth, so brace yourself!** Net profit is, I believe, by far the most significant number for any business. (Nothing else much matters if a company isn't profitable.) Production, collection, new patients seen, units of crown and bridge completed can all be useful data. But it is disappointing that this crucial figure of net is the one fact never disclosed in so much of what passes for practice management literature. I believe serious students of the business of dentistry deserve better.

I'm intensely cognizant of the cultural indelicacy of discussing net income (and obviously severely intimidated by a combination of low self-esteem and this taboo), but without being privy to the ultimate bottom line, how can one accurately evaluate the true usefulness of any business system or scheme? It seems to me crucial, if I am determined to shoot my mouth off concerning business-related topics, that readers be apprised of all key facts.

My insecurity salved, to the greatest extent possible, let's get to it. By age 40 I had a million dollars in savings. I don't mean my net worth was a million, including office, home, cars, furniture, clothes, pets, gold fillings, etc. I'm referring to having no debt, while owning stocks, bonds, mutual funds and money market funds totaling this amount.

By this time, income from my investments exceeded our family-of-six cost of living. (Megan and Rachel had joined and completed the "firm"--unless one counts grandson Hunter John Ubbe Wilde.) **I'd achieved my dream of financial freedom -- after working my way through school, and starting an office without a single patient--after 12 years of private practice.**

I also entered a treatment center for alcoholics that year. To this once-indigent boy's utter stupefaction, it seemed money really couldn't buy happiness! I began therapy the morning of the day my darling, then five-year-old daughter, Megan, was admitted to the same hospital. She'd suffered a brain injury and fractured skull, then lapsed into a coma. (All this damage was the result of losing a dispute with a four-wheeler that held a significant weight advantage.)

Meg has recovered completely, and is in her junior year of college. I haven't had one drink of alcohol in over 14 years. (All the gory details of my addiction and Meg's injury are recorded in the introduction of *Dentistry's Future*, for those who are interested. It was a helpful, if painful, exercise to write about such a pivotal period of my life. Any reader who feels I'm guilty of grandiosity--a familiar AA word--in my unfailingly candid discussion of personal and professional finance, should be placated by reading that account of my destruction and rebirth.)

Nothing in my life has rewarded me as greatly as my, to date at least, successful battle with alcoholism. I'm still far short of the person I'd like to be, but I've grown as an individual and a dentist by facing this implacable foe. As a result of that growth, I've achieved a modicum of wisdom and joy. My other dental books contained lengthy passages dealing with the essential topic of creating a philosophy of joy. No subject fills me with greater excitement, or, I feel, is more meaningful. But in this book, I'll reluctantly limit myself to the following few comments concerning this crucial issue.

I have proven to myself--the hard way--that there can be **no success without happiness.** Now, there's a lesson many dentists badly need to ingest, as did I some 14 years ago. I lived the famous short story, "The Monkey's Paw" (either you know it or you don't), achieving my version of what I thought to be success--to my horror--and survived.

No matter how lucrative one's practice, if one is not happy about and excited by one's existence, that dentist is failing. As my sagacious friend, Dr. Paddi Lund, said in his extraordinary book, *Building the Happiness Centered Business,* trading misery at the office to earn money to try to buy happiness elsewhere is a fool's bargain.

You can purchase this great book, from this splendid Australian dentist, by calling *Private Practice,* the excellent and unusual newsletter published by Dr. Barry Polansky, at 800-453-9891. Barry is Paddi's good friend and is privileged to distribute all Dr. Lund's products here "in the states."

Paddi's book is easy to read, inspirational and filled with insights to enable anyone to become a better person, and better dental care provider. I couldn't recommend reading it more highly! While you're on the phone, you might see if Barry would part with a free issue of *Private Practice* for your perusal. If you enjoy my book, or Paddi's, I think you'll be very excited by the content of this innovative newsletter.

Another example of a foundational truth I've learned: **wisdom consists of accurate knowledge that is ACTED UPON.** No benefit accrues from erudition that is never employed. In fact, having correct information one doesn't utilize is anything but wise. For example, it will do no good to memorize this book, if those efforts don't result in your implementing changes (acting) to improve your office in ways that will increase profits, and improve the circumstances of patients and staff.

Completing three weeks in a treatment center, and enduring three days and two nights without sleep while Megan remained in her coma, had given me a great deal of time, and a powerful motivation, to rethink the core precepts of my existence. Given my agonizing circumstances at that time, I was pretty sure something basic had gone awry. Financial freedom hadn't proven quite the blessing a person who grew up in poverty had expected.

But, here's the key....**I acted on my hard-won wisdom!** I slowed my practice down, hired associates, and quit worrying about money. (Don't misunderstand. I still very much LIKE money, probably due to so many years of existence when it was in such short supply. But I'd never make a decision today based on money considerations alone.)

None of the goals I'd set for myself--the practice, high net worth, or positive community regard--and for which I'd worked so hard and sacrificed so much to achieve, had provided me with lasting peace or joy. (And there can be no success without joy.)

I began a deliberate effort--one I've never ceased--to get to know and understand myself. To honestly perceive the wonderful and pathetic creature I am, and to grow to accept, then love myself. To consciously and perpetually strive to create a life that, for me, was joyously fulfilling, resting firmly on a bedrock of accurate self-awareness. Every such journey is unique, but, for purposes of illustration, allow me to offer a glimpse of my path.

I started writing; something which, for reasons I can't explain, I deeply love. I write four to five hours every day possible, and resent the days I can't. Due far more to diligence than talent, I've had seven books--five dental--and over 100 articles published.

I started hunting every moment I could, as in hunting I find my truest passion and most complete fulfillment. I played more tennis and racquetball, expanded my garden, began to enjoy frequent long and exotic family vacations. In short, I began doing things I really liked, and avoiding things--like exhausting days of providing dental care--I disliked. (Shouldn't we all be trying to do this, as much as possible, anyway? Doesn't doing what one enjoys, while avoiding the unpleasant, seem an obvious step on one's journey to happiness? And isn't this manifest truth damn hard for a dentist to achieve?)

But consider this major point, more directly related to most reader's goals. In the office, reduced treatment hours allowed me to focus even more on profitability through **SYSTEM REFINEMENT**. Working smarter, not harder, as such efforts are often described. I like doing things well--it makes me feel good--and have enjoyed some success in this regard.

Please allow me to share some of the rewards forthcoming from perpetual and intelligent **system refinements**. As an example, in 1996 I saw patients a total of 52 eight-hour days, and had a **net income from dentistry alone of $347,000**. That's a **DAILY NET OF $6,673**, over 13 times the 1994 ADA statistical average of $480 per day. (To be thorough, my investment income that year was $338,600. I can't take much credit for this outstanding fiscal result, as I'm smart enough not to confuse genius with a bull market. A major portion of these well-performing investment assets were sequestered in my retirement plan, but still, you should have seen the 1996 tax bill! The Tax Reform Act of 1986 KILLED small businesses.)

The keys to achieving such profitability involved employing associate dentists, and constantly enhancing office systems, none more critical to our success than our very profitable hygiene department. (Never fear, you'll get to peruse every statistic I monitor concerning our hygiene results, during the course of this book. And I monitor damn near everything imaginable!)

I sold my practice and retired in May, 2000, at age 53. I even let my dental (not hunting!) license lapse. I believe dentists who love their work are the most blessed people on this earth. I devoutly wish I could claim membership in their ranks. But dentistry has always been extremely difficult and very stressful for me.

When I decided to retire, neither of my associates wished to purchase my practice. Both eventually relocated to become employees in other offices. I worked as a solo provider the last 10 months of my career, after 15 years as owner of a small group practice where I had provided patient care only one or two days a week. And I do mean work! I don't know how you guys and gals in full-time solo practice do it!

The only positive forthcoming from that 10 months--other than very significant profits--was my complete certainty that I was wise to quit, and the knowledge that I'd never even vaguely consider practicing again.

So, there you have a brief glimpse of my history, from birth to the moment of this writing. I hope this background will provide insight to help you understand the reasoning behind many of my decisions, revealed in the course of this document. As we proceed to discuss hygiene, I promise a factual description, detailing only and exactly what I've already accomplished, not some science-fiction pipedream of dental hygiene utopia.

I want you to clearly comprehend what we accomplished in our hygiene department--the exact results and precisely how we achieved them--working in a predominantly middle-class community of 13,000 that contains nine dentists. For, as one of my heroes, Dr. Omer Reed, has asserted, "If something's already been done, chances are it's possible."

Why Hygiene?

There are three major reasons why I'm writing a book primarily dedicated to dental hygiene management and enhancement.

1. I get an average of two to three calls per week from dentists wishing to discuss something I've written. At least **50 percent of those inquiries deal with hygiene.** Far more than any other subject among the broad panoply of topics I address.
2. My friend, mentor and ex-boss, Dr. Woody Oakes (I was assistant editor with Woody's *The Profitable Dentist* newsletter for a year or so, and still contribute an occasional article), has advised me that any lectures, video or audio tapes he offers about hygiene are always best-sellers. Nobody knows more about dentists' interests than Woody. (Few know as much about anything as the unassuming, but omniscient Dr. Oakes.) Both Woody's and my experience indicate **the demand for information concerning hygiene is high.**

   When I began to research this work, I called the ADA Library. I asked their wonderful staff to send me any book ever published dealing with the MANAGEMENT of a dental hygiene department. After a thorough search--and these are thorough and dedicated folks--they called me back and said they could find no book ever written on the subject. **The supply of information concerning optimal hygiene administration is low.** (Until now!)

3. In addition to my Economics 101 awareness of the significance of high demand and low supply, I believe hygiene to be the least efficiently employed segment of our inexact profession. (I don't mean to brag, but when it comes to creating inefficiency, dentistry is hard to beat. Being considered the least efficient segment of a hard-working but frequently incompetent profession is no mean feat!)

Being poorly run means the upside for hygiene is tremendous! All that untapped potential (and since our office has "tapped" this vein for many years, I know what "acres of diamonds" lie hidden beneath) makes highly profitable hygiene a very exciting topic. I believe the average dental practice can greatly increase the effectiveness of the periodontal therapy they offer, thus enhancing their patients' health, improving staff compensation and enjoyment, while being well rewarded financially for this excellent achievement.

Making all facets of the above statement come true, for inspired dental offices, is my primary motivation in writing this book.

Allow me to digress with the first of what I hope will be many asides. (People tell me such ramblings are usually the best parts of the book .... I'm uncertain precisely how one should evaluate such a seemingly left-handed compliment.)

I listened to an audio tape recently, in which a successful dentist, from a major metropolitan area, explained the key to his achievements was performing only procedures he really enjoyed, and at which he excelled. His well-intentioned advice to all dentists was to concentrate their efforts on what they do best. I believe there is some truth to this assertion. For example, I hated removing teeth, and seldom did. This reduced my stress, and freed me to perform more satisfying, and often profitable, procedures.

But I practice in a blue-collar community, where families of four to six members typically subsisted on an annual income of $40,000 or less. Even with thousands of patients from which to choose, I had to work for a living! I'm sure I never completed a $5,000 case in my career! There are no veneerodontists or implantalogists working full-time in our frugal area. We provided pedo, perio, endo, fixed and removable pros, operative, ortho and TMJ care in our office.

Here's a first, even for me: an aside within an aside. I fabricated an average of two hard mouth-guards a week. So many patients suffered from TMJ symptoms, sensitive cervical abrasion and abfraction lesions, extreme wear or fractures of tooth and restoration, that the need for such appliances was quite high.

I believe skillfully crafted, hard mouth-guards can eliminate discomfort and prevent damage to dental health. Such mouth-guards are a wonderful service, and, with the help of a **fine system,** their fabrication can prove to be very profitable. (The brilliant Dr. Gordon Christensen, who seems to know a lot about such matters, has made numerous statements concerning the enormous need of patients for such mouth-guards.)

The study models and bites (centric and protrusive) needed to create a mouth-guard were usually taken by my hygiene assistant. My lab technician, Mr. Larry Robbins, who has been creating excellent removable dental appliances since 1963, fabricated the mouth-guards, and did the preliminary intra-oral fit and bite adjusting.

Other than discussing the need and function of a mouth-guard during exams, my total time involved in the entire process was 10 minutes, scheduled to refine the occlusion. Since Larry is damn good at such adjustments, I usually had about 5 minutes of the appointment remaining for a quick cup of coffee.

According to Connie, the insurance expert in my former office, my lab cost for this appliance was $65. The fee we charged (ADA code 9940) was $289. This means our office made a net profit of ($289 - $65 =) $224. Since total doctor time involved was 1/6th of an hour (10 minutes), hourly NET was (6 x $224 =) **$1,344 net/hour.**

I know this rough calculation doesn't include any overhead but the lab bill; however--for those not bothering to treat occlusal problems--it ought to include some real food for thought. Take a minute and calculate similar net figures for a crown or denture. Just subtract lab cost from one's fee, then divide by total dentist time scheduled for the procedure. I promise you'll learn something valuable from the exercise.

(Okay, I'll help just this once. For illustration purposes, assume a crown fee of $600 and a lab bill of $100. Crown net after lab is $600 - $100 = $500. If 80 minutes of doctor time is required to prep and seat the restoration, the net per hour is $500 / 1.33 hours = $376 net/hour. It's also much more demanding to fabricate excellent fixed restorations (and one is much more exposed to possible unfortunate predicaments) than it is to make a mouth-guard. My last clue: $376 is LESS than $1,344.)

I thus end my aside (aside), and return (seamlessly?) to my first digression, concerning the wisdom of limiting one's efforts to areas where he or she already possesses significant skills. I contend there is little upside remaining concerning things one already does well, but tremendous growth potential involving procedures for which one is, at least at the moment, not especially skilled.

Consider this: I love tennis, and play as much as my aging body allows. If I worked hard--conditioned, played often, took lessons-I could enhance my game...a little.

I played some golf, about 30 years ago. The game made my teeth ache, so I gave it up. If I play a round to establish a base score (I'm certain the score would be base), then began to take lessons, faithfully worked at the driving range, got in 18 holes a day, etc., I could quickly improve my skills, I'd guess by a significant amount. (I don't wish to brag, but with hard work and time, I feel confident I could elevate my game from dreadful to pathetic. Hey, I'm an athlete!)

Do you make mouth-guards? Have you tried the amazingly effective new, automated endodontic techniques? How profitable is your hygiene department? Ever considered orthodontics--which I performed for 15 years? (And where parents beg you to take their thousands of dollars, and give little Amanda a beautiful smile!) Maybe doing just what one enjoys isn't the complete answer for every dentist and every situation. I mean, how much can you realistically expect to enhance your skill, efficiency and productivity taking another C & B course?

Where the hell was I? Oh yes, the upside of hygiene. (I heard that "finally!") Here's why I am pretty sure my ideas can help most practices. According to the May, 1998, *Dental Economics* practice survey, the average hygienist produced $6,835 per month, or (12 x $6,835 =) $82,020 per year. *Dental Economics* didn't break the figures down beyond this point, but if one assumes a 40-hour week, that calculated to a productivity of approximately $43 per hour. ($6,835 / 160 hours = $43 per hour.)

I've practiced all my career employing just one full-time hygienist at a time. In 1999, my wonderful hygienist, Melissa Lannery, R.D.H., produced $173,270. This total was somewhat attenuated by lost days due to only one dentist (me) working in the office, but was still almost identical to her 1998 total of $173,783--both years fairly typical for our practice. Her 1999 hourly average production was $133--almost **three times the national average.** ($133 / $43 = 3).

We'll share our numbers for the entire year of 1999 in great detail later, but I thought I'd offer a tidbit of our achievements, to whet the old appetite, or at least keep you reading. Melissa tripled the national average for hourly production, but since most hygiene expenses are fixed (salary being by far the biggest investment) the **increase in my net hygiene profit was MUCH GREATER THAN 300 percent, as we'll examine later.**

I've used the same basic system of expanded hygiene, with gradual refinements, for about 15 years. Seven dentists--myself included--have overseen our periodontal department over that period of years. I've employed four hygienists over that time and God alone knows how many other staff. Throughout, our profits and production have remained outstanding. Melissa is the best hygienist I've ever worked with--one of my heroes in dentistry and life--but **it's the system, not the people, that accounts for our success.**

In this book I'm offering readers a detailed look at hygiene, a system that is possibly 400 to 500 percent more profitable than average. In what other foundation areas of your practice do you believe productivity can be so greatly enhanced? (It's not fair to count starting to fabricate mouth-guards!)

Here are my goals for this book. These are also the objectives that I suggest every reader should have achieved once he or she has mastered and implemented the material within.

1. I will offer directions so complete and concise they will allow any motivated dentist to **establish a highly efficient and profitable hygiene department, based on this single resource**. I'll

do my best to answer all your questions, before you can ask them.

2. I'll help you and your team achieve **consistent delivery of the highest level of periodontal service** your ability, knowledge, and effort make possible.

   Mouth-guards are a valuable service, but optional. I believe every office should offer state-of-the-art periodontal care to all patients. Healthy periodontium is the footing upon which all oral fitness rests, and as our profession and the public are discovering more fully every day, is also critical to over-all systemic health.

3. By employing our hygiene system, one's **overall practice net profit should increase dramatically**. Of course, hygiene will be much more lucrative, but powerful ideas will be offered to enhance patient flow, and thus increase the number of recare exams performed. This increased patient volume will act as a gas pedal, accelerating one's entire office financial situation. (I'll also offer some thoughts as to how one might increase new patients and meaningfully enhance the new patient examination experience, thus improving case acceptance levels, and a whole lot more.)

4. **Staff will grow closer,** united by a common bond of pride and satisfaction achieved from knowing they are offering excellence, while enjoying the appreciation patients show for this unusual level of service.

5. **One's practice will expand overall,** as excellence--so uncommon today -- is always rewarded. Demographics--increasing population, high employment, record-setting economy and level of affluence, juxtaposed with a declining number of dentists--make this a propitious time for any dental practice to pur-

sue aggressive growth. (I'd also keep this thought in mind: Good times don't last forever. **I'd strongly suggest one strike while the iron is still hot!**)

It's impossible to keep true excellence a secret! The truth will out, and patients will flock to your door, demanding your services. There is little in life I've discovered more satisfying than the quiet awareness that one is offering the best, and being fully and fairly rewarded emotionally and financially, as is commensurate with such an exceptional accomplishment.

Increased quality of service, increased joy, increased profit, increased self-esteem, increased practice profile and reputation, increased net worth (significantly).... For obtaining all these desirable objectives, one will be rewarded by life more abundantly. **The awareness of a job well done, and enjoying the richly rewarding fruits of one's honestly earned achievements, are critical to attaining something for which I can attach no specific value, price or title, but that may be called peace.**

****

SEGMENT I

ESTABLISHING PROFITABLE DENTAL HYGIENE

Chapter 1

An Examination of the Current Dentist/Hygienist Situation

(Although expanded and totally rewritten, some portions of Chapters 1 through 4 contain information first introduced in Chapter 5 of *Dentistry's Future*. Such repetition will occur periodically throughout this book, and will be clearly noted. Rewriting previously published information allows me to update previous work, and lets this text serve as a stand-alone resource, providing almost everything one ever needs to know--or at least everything I know--concerning profitable dental hygiene.)

We are about to examine the concepts and workings of an excellent hygiene department, using my practice as our primary model and point of reference. Performing hygiene in the manner we'll scrutinize will:

1. Be highly profitable for the practice owner(s).
2. Allow the best possible clinical care to be provided for every patient.

3. Decrease the customary frustration, boredom and drudgery inherent to providing periodontal therapy, while greatly enhancing possible hygienist remuneration.
4. Allow skilled staff to invest an extra 20 minutes with each hygiene patient. This time should be devoted to patient education and relationship building, thus proving to be of immense value to one's dental practice.

Please consider the primary contention upon which this book rests: **No modern office can achieve its optimal potential without having a highly PROFITABLE hygiene department!! NONE!!!** Conversely, the finest possible practice, functioning without hygiene, can be enhanced if a superb periodontal program is added.

Contemporary standards of care mandate competent treatment of every patient's periodontal tissues. Possessing the skills and offering the effort to restore every patient's mouth to optimal periodontal health is a must.

As we touched on in the introduction, dental hygiene exemplifies vast potential, frequently juxtaposed with disappointing results and thus enormous conflict and distress for all parties involved. **In no other area of our profession is the typical dentist's lack of business acumen more glaringly apparent, or a viable option to enhance fiscal return more readily available.** Hygiene represents a rich vein of ore over which most dental offices camp unawares, not even attempting to sift nuggets with their fingers from the fecund dust below their feet.

As I've mentioned, I speak with dentists frequently concerning a variety of matters (too damn few of which involve hunting). No topic generates more interest, or more emotion, than the subject of hygiene. The complaints and concerns I most often hear include:

Dentists' Concerns with Hygiene

1. Hygiene loses money.

A dear friend of mine went through an excellent and extensive one-day course offered by noted practice management expert Dr. Charles Blair. His entire office numbers were analyzed to the most minute level, employing Dr. Blair's sophisticated software and superb personal expertise.

(Dr. Blair and his associates can be reached by calling 704-424-9780. They offer a fine newsletter, excellent courses and myriad services that are a real boon to any dentist who wishes to be a better business manager and thus enjoy enhanced profits.)

At the time of Dr. Blair's review, my friend's office employed five hygienists. This dental entrepreneur extraordinaire (the day of this writing, his staff totaled 49) was horrified to find he was **losing approximately $5 per prophy**! That's a bite, when one's staff performs around 40 prophys a day, or 200 per week! (Two hundred prophys per week at -$5 = $1,000 loss per week, or **$50,000 loss from hygiene alone per year!**)

Once he became aware of the undeniable reality of his hygiene situation, quick and decisive steps were immediately implemented. But, before the aid of Dr. Blair's data, my gifted and astute friend had no idea how much his hygiene department was draining office revenue.

Mercifully, most dentists don't have sufficient patients or staff to allow them to lose money at that accelerated rate. As a matter of fact, few dentists with whom I've spoken even know with certainty if their office makes a profit, or suffers a loss, from hygiene. (Every reader will be able to clearly, easily and irrefutably make that vital determination before finishing this book.)

If the hygienist's production is greater than his or her salary, is one doing okay? Sure...unless the hygienist is treating patients IN YOUR OFFICE, and thus there exists significant overhead expense, in addition to salary, with which one must cope. But let's reserve a detailed discussion concerning the calculation of overhead and profit in hygiene until later.

At this juncture, suffice it to say many dentists consider hygiene as a money-losing, time-eating, pain-in-the-rump, necessary-evil segment of their practice. And most sadly, for many offices, this correctly describes the current reality. (This description of a fictional hygiene department is weirdly similar to how I would describe a long-ago girl friend!) But, as I'm about to illustrate clearly, **it doesn't have to be that way!**

2. Hygienists' attitudes can be less than ideal.

In a significant portion of our nation, hygienists are in short supply, thus great demand. This is sure as hell true in most small rural communities of the Midwest, and has been FOREVER! (Or, at least for the increasingly significant portion of forever of which I'm aware.)

I personally know of excellent offices--thank the Good Lord, not mine--which have invested YEARS and significant revenue in their efforts to employ a hygienist. We'll consider recruiting hygienists shortly, but allow me to note that--while I've never had to practice a total of more than a few weeks during my entire career without benefit of a hygienist's critical services--it's been a decade since my most diligent search efforts were able to attract more than a single potential hygienist employee. (Interviewing under such circumstances is like hunting all day for one shot. When you finally get an opportunity, you'd better BEAR DOWN!)

This supply/demand relationship can create an inversion, where the potential hygienist-employee is, in fact, in charge. I've often interviewed hygienists who had multiple job offers already on the table, while he or she was the only applicant our office had been able to attract. And both of us were aware of this reality. (While only half of us was pleased about it!)

Under such circumstances, I've always been acutely aware that, despite the office bearing my name, and my being the party offering salary and benefits, I am the one being interviewed. I'm pleased to report that I've been able to hire every hygienist to whom I offered a position. Our success in this critical endeavor partly relates to our excellent general office appearance, and particularly to our fine hygiene physical facilities.

Our hygiene area consists of two large, attractively decorated operatories, with excellent, modern units. Each room features every device I can think of--x-ray head, computer terminal, nitrous oxide plumbed to each, intra-oral camera connected to cable television, virtual reality glasses, piezo-scalers--anything to enhance our hygienist's abilities to offer state-of-the-art care in as much comfort as is humanly possible to create. Offering every conceivable physical advantage is essential to successful recruitment, but also imperative to providing the best possible periodontal care for one's patients, while maximizing staff comfort and hygiene profitability.

We also have job candidates review our documented history of outstanding production, and thus exceptional compensation, of previous hygienists in our office, going back a decade or more. The physical setting and factual history (broken down into average hygienist compensation per hour), accurately demonstrate our profound commitment to providing the best possible care under as close to ideal conditions as possible. (It sure ain't my good looks or charm that gets hygienists to commit to our office! It's more like, in spite of, or so my loyal staff assures me.)

Returning to the subject of troubling attitudes, over the course of my career, I've often been asked by hygienists to chat with them at day's end. Such requests frequently precipitated icy sweats and violent shakes. I knew they had some complaint or request, both similar in that they always caused me trouble and cost me money. I also understood that, whatever their demands--and I've heard some dillies--I had little choice but to grin and nod my head yes.

Let's cut to the chase. I pay all salaries, and it is my name on the office door, but in the small portion of the planet where I reside, if push comes to shove, no matter the hygienist's skills or attitude, both of us know the hygienist could be working in another office the following week, while I'd be extremely fortunate to replace her in a month! It was always the case that I needed her more than she needed me, and we both knew it. (If I lapse into the female pronoun on occasion, forgive me. I've had only one male staff member, he for a total of about three months, during my entire career. I've grown accustomed to thinking of my team members as "she.")

(Our current wonderful hygienist, Melissa Lannery, R.D.H., nicknamed "Sunshine," was a joy and blessing to our office. She never abused her power, or made a single request not motivated by her desire to provide ideal patient care. I consider her to be the epitome of professionalism, and am frequently embarrassed by how short of her lofty standards in attitude and ability I fall. Bear in mind that I'm retired, and no longer have to be nice to anyone. I wish to acknowledge that it was an honor and privilege to spend the final four-plus years of my career working with Melissa!)

More typically than the above heartfelt paean, when dentists discuss hygienists, I hear expressions such as "prima donna," he or she acts like they are too good for the rest of the team, is disruptive, won't make an effort to fit in, is self-centered...you get the idea. (While we dentists are SO WELL ADJUSTED!)

3. Hygiene is perceived as a disrupter of the day and **a drag on the dentist's production.**

Performing hygiene recare examinations is not consistently listed among the top 5,000 favorite pastimes of the average dentist. (Hygiene checks usually fall slightly below "being poked in the eye with a sharp stick," on dentists' hierarchy of joys.) Lengthy, complex, demanding treatment is frequently forced to be interrupted because of hygiene checks. And if the examination is not conducted promptly, the dentist must often face the gimlet-eyed glare of a behind-schedule-and-not-happy-about-it-because-it's-all-your-fault! hygienist. (Brrrr!)

All realize such interruptions are not the hygienist's fault, as his or her professionalism, office policy and patient needs demand timeliness. But it's tiring for dentists to have to run this circuit of recall checks every day. (In my dreams, this endless running from room to room, while being haunted by ghosts of hygienists past, is roughly equivalent to Dante's eighth circle of hell!)

The frustration of being forced to interrupt treatment, seemingly at the worst possible moment, combined with the fact that one need not have an MBA to realize the examinations one abandoned his or her eight-veneer case three times to perform are nowhere near as profitable as fine restorative dental care, results in a mental state for many dentists far to the left of Nirvana.

(As we'll see in a bit, expanded hygiene allows at least a 20-minute window of opportunity during which the dentist may examine the patient at any time without interrupting or delaying one's hygienist.)

4. Hygiene is seen as a disproportionate drain on staff effort, and a primary cause of office overload and stress.

Keeping a hygiene schedule fully booked requires a great deal of staff time. Many dentists wonder if this energy would not be more wisely invested in public relations, checking on insurance questions, or any other activity resulting in maximizing the dentist's production. The lower one's hygienist's productivity, the more pressing this question becomes.

Assisting hygiene patients with scheduling, payment and insurance, and myriad other miscellaneous concerns at the end of their treatment adds stress to the front desk, crowds the reception room and generally pushes the office toward unpleasant overload, all for the reward of what is too frequently a seemingly minor, if not negative, remuneration.

Other considerations remain, but I think one can grasp the idea inherent within these basic four. In short, many dentists are frustrated and discouraged with the status of hygiene, as it currently exists, in too many modern dental offices.

Most dentists realize they don't possess the periodontal skills equivalent to an excellent hygienist's. Most don't really want to. The majority of dentists with whom I am acquainted would rather be poked in the (insert an anatomical location of maximum personal motivation) with a sharp scaler than be forced to spend even one eight-hour day cleaning teeth!

Within our profession's current 60+ percent overhead world, aware dentists also realize they can't afford to reduce time devoted to restorative care to personally perform the relatively low-production task of cleaning teeth. Thus dentists and patients desperately need the valuable services of hygienists, despite the above-listed concerns.

Hygiene's Concerns with Dentistry

Don't believe for a second, doctor, that frustration concerning hygiene is a one-way street, or you may be trampled by traffic headed in the opposite direction. Hygienists also have expressed numerous valid concerns or complaints about the dentist-hygienist relationship as it exists most commonly today.

I read PennWell Publishing's fine *RDH Magazine* carefully each month. The editor, Mark Hartley, is a superb professional, excellent writer, and a friend. I've written for his publication several times. I receive *RDH*, as I like to remain abreast of what's happening in the world of hygiene, as it represents an integral portion of my practice's success.

I believe most dentists would be amazed by the controversy, unrest and naked anger openly displayed toward dentists and the dental profession in some of this splendid magazine's articles. There is a very vocal segment (I have no idea of their numbers, but the pointed rhetoric is powerful and perpetual) who consider organized dentistry as the enemy, and are dedicated and determined to struggle valiantly to "throw off the shackles of dentist oppression," and enhance the autonomy of the hygiene profession.

I'm a vocal proponent of hygiene, and of the valuable, honorable and skilled members of this profession, but as a dentist, I'm obviously not whom hygiene would choose to be their spokesperson.

So, let me clearly state, I have no authority or mandate to speak on behalf of hygienists. Given my lack of access to hygiene's inner circle and deepest thoughts (my opinions being based mainly on personal experience and the many articles I've read), my perception of their complaint is that being controlled by dental boards and dentists stifles opportunities to independently define their profession, and truncates growth and income potential. The expressed contention is so bitter, I believe many hygienists feel a significant number of dentists perceive them to be their personal enemies.

As periodic state elections to legalize independent hygiene indicate, a very real problem exists within the current dentist-hygienist relationship, at least on the national or macro level. (I know of many individual situations, similar to our office, where the association between hygienist and dentist working together is one of mutual respect and affection. It's often the "other" dentists with whom hygienists have problems.)

I've read articles from both dentists and hygienists concerning the cause, and possible solutions, to this raw interface that damages and embarrasses both professions. There are many suggestions extant to ameliorate these problems, ranging from hygienists functioning independently of dentists, to in-office preceptor programs replacing hygiene schools (perceived by hygienists as a dagger held to their throat), to group psychotherapy of the Rodney King, "Can't we all just get along?" school of thought.

Most of the proposed solutions contain some merit, but--as the conflicts' continued festering during the three decades of my career indicates--are merely ineffectually hacking at the leaves of the dilemma. I wish to advance a bold proposal to the profession that strikes to the root of this conundrum.

I contend the basic cause of the dentist-versus-hygienist conflict is fiscal in nature. As we discuss optimizing hygiene, consider for yourself what portion of existing distress results from financial disappointments of hygienists and dentists alike. Or how a 50 percent increase in your hygienist's compensation, and a similar 50 percent increase in hygiene NET for the dentist, might influence all parties' perceptions of reality. (A 50 percent raise--a MINIMUM GOAL for expanded hygiene--is a soothing balm for most business strife.)

The ultimate solution to a financially based problem lies, not in identifying clever ways to slice the existing asset pie to everyone's satisfaction, but in establishing a system that makes more abundant revenue (a bigger pie) available for all parties. And that is precisely what profitable expanded hygiene accomplishes.

I don't believe it behooves our profession to vegetate and watch this unseemly strife continue. By law in most states, the dentist is the business owner, so it is incumbent upon the doctor to devise a plan to enhance hygiene income and improve relationships of all parties involved. (To eliminate confusion, if one's name appears on the bottom right line of paychecks, like it or not, he or she is the responsible party.)

Being the party that creates a mutually agreeable resolution keeps dentists proactive. Creating a win-win solution seems a much better employment of energy than sporadically fighting independent hygiene bills, or firmly placing our fingers in our collective ears, humming loudly, ignoring problems as much as possible, and just hoping everything works out. (The above delineated approach represents my recollection of suggested staff management techniques circa 1972, University of Iowa, College of Dentistry. I tried this approach early in my career, but had trouble fixing teeth without taking my fingers out of my ear-holes. Also, staff can always throw things, if they really want your attention.)

A proposed solution to the dentist-hygienist problems will be forthcoming based on sound business principles, and increased awareness that both dentist's and hygienist's times are rare and valuable commodities. Thus any effort or fiscal contribution that serves to enhance the productivity of hygienists represents a potentially positive and valuable investment to all parties involved.

If a system can be established that:

1. is extraordinarily profitable for dental practices,
2. ends the hygienist shortage instantly,
3. allows hygienists to be significantly better compensated, while enhancing their working environment,
4. while providing a superior quality of clinical care for every patient--we'll have established a rare and difficult accomplishment--a win/win/win scenario. Such an enlightened office, basking in the glow of this triumphant achievement, will enjoy the serenity bequeathed by a mind-set of mutual abundance, not divisive scarcity.

Dentists can't afford to WIN this professional battle. Hygienists' services are too integral to our profession's success to allow them to suffer such a defeat. Only ending the dentist/hygienist tumult with mutual success for all parties will allow the formation of an ideal team.

The above-listed four goals describe the dentist-hygienist universe in which I choose to reside. Please allow the thoughts that follow to serve as my personal invitation for all who so desire to join me in this superior world. The necessary ticket is an understanding (wisdom) and implementation (power) of the concept of **profitable expanded hygiene.**

Chapter 2

The Mechanism of Expanded Hygiene

Enough of the philosophic overview concerning current hygienist/dentist relationships and proposed general suggestions to improve same. It's helpful to understand the basic underpinnings of a situation, but my typical desire is to jump directly to the heart of any conundrum. So let's begin to develop a definitive answer to the problems so far addressed.

I contend the system of expanded hygiene that my practice enjoyed for 15 years offers the ideal solution to all the previous discussed concerns of dentists and hygienists. If that is the case, it would behoove one to carefully study how such an advantaged strategy operates. So let's consider a typical day of expanded hygiene.

Our office day begins 20 minutes before our first patient is scheduled, with the entire staff meeting in the lab, gathered around that day's master schedule, for our morning huddle and clearing. (We post copies of our schedule in all operatories, but the master schedule is where any changes that occur during the day are recorded. After our meeting, this day-sheet is taped to the hallway wall that everyone passes on the way to the treatment areas.)

Either the night before, or earlier that morning, I have reviewed the records of my scheduled patients, as well as those to be seen in hygiene that day. I've noted on the master schedule what x-rays are required that day (something only a dentist may diagnose), and any unusual matters--as past problems or complaints (last visit, sensitivity #3 area to cold), specific materials needed for today's care (we'll use Impergum for this partial impression), or uncompleted treatment of which we need to be aware. (A bridge was recommended to replace #30. Do we have insurance information?)

Melissa will have also reviewed her patient records, and made notes--perhaps where pockets were deepest, areas of sensitivity, patient refuses fluoride, or wishes to not lie back too far--on her separate hygiene schedule.

With the entire staff present, we discuss each patient to be seen that day, noting the unusual. While Melissa and I have done the research, the entire team may contribute. Chairsides might help us by mentioning that a patient suffers from a severe gag reflex. Front office people might caution of a potential payment problem, and request we do no other treatment than what is scheduled that day. A divorce, family illness, new baby, recent vacation...might be mentioned to get us all up to speed, and allow more personalization of the patient visit. This entire process takes about five minutes.

It requires about 40 minutes of my time to review all records, and I've grown damn tired of the process. But I've always found the knowledge I glean to be worth far more than my investment of time. I crave a well-run, timely office, and this beginning is an integral portion of my consistently achieving such a desired result.

Just being aware of each patient's complete treatment plan

(what's scheduled that day, and also treatment planned for future visits) often allows me to fill holes that appear in that day's schedule, by performing additional care on an already appointed patient. (For example, if I was told an hour had opened later in the morning, I'd have the option of preparing my current patient's two lower left molars for crowns, instead of the single upper right tooth scheduled.)

This benefit of reviewing records alone has results in thousands of dollars of increased production each year. It also reduces my frustration, as I hate having the rhythm of a pleasant day disrupted by a break in the schedule, and after sitting around for half an hour, I tend to lose all my momentum.

At the end of this patient treatment review, we hold our clearing. This is an opportunity to advise teammates of one's emotional status. If all is well, and one is prepared to contribute 100 percent for the day, simply stating "I'm clear" will suffice.

But some days one of the team is feeling a little less than completely intact. Knowing of a sore throat or upset stomach allows us to provide needed support to our ailing friend. This is vastly superior to being unaware of a problem, and becoming frustrated by a team member who is a "bit off" that day, while in fact, she is heroically working under less than optimal conditions, willing to suffer distress to support her co-workers and boss.

Emotional concerns, such as the illness of a child or loved one, can also cause distractions. Again, awareness allows us to offer succor. Some days I'm the one that is troubled. But even on my best days, I need all the help I can get from every member of my team. If I wish for their support, I must freely and fully give of mine.

I lead this huddle and clearing. The tone of the day will be set by this first brief time a staff spends together. **A grumpy dentist in the morning will have a grumpy staff that day.** Doctor, if you are only going to be pleasant 10 minutes over a given 24-hour period, try your best to have this blessed event occur during this critical morning meeting!

Clear as to our duties for the day, and emotionally bonded as a team, we are ready to begin offering care. Let's peek over Melissa's shoulder, and observe expanded hygiene in action.

Expanded Hygiene

Expanded hygiene requires two rooms, and a full-time chair-side assistant, totally dedicated to hygiene. Let's consider how a typical day employing such a system would proceed.

As our hygienist is treating her first patient of the day in Room 1, her assistant seats the next hygiene patient in the second room that she has previously prepared.

The hygiene assistant exposes any already dentist-diagnosed x-rays (that I've noted on the schedule), helps the patient review and update his medical history (this updated medical history is initialed and dated by the patient), and takes a blood pressure reading, if indicated. The assistant makes certain the patient is comfortable, while spending a few moments establishing rapport and answering questions. (For long appointments, such as the C, D, and F level of soft tissue care we'll describe shortly, the assistant provides the patient with a warmed, herbal-scented neck pillow, heated for 90 seconds in our microwave.)

When the hygienist completes her portion of care for the first patient, she shifts to the second room where the next patient awaits, already draped and reclined, with the above-listed tasks completed. All instrumentation and equipment is ready, and Melissa can immediately wash her hands, don gloves and begin performing therapy.

The assistant moves to the first room where she notifies the dentist, through our intercom system, that "the patient in Room 1 is ready for his **first check**." She then polishes, flosses, and administers topical fluoride (if law allows in your state). If so instructed by the hygienist, she reviews oral hygiene and demonstrates any recommended dental health aids (flossing aids, bridge cleaners, Rota-dent® brush, etc.).

Often, intra-oral camera images have been suggested, and are exposed by the assistant. These may have been requested during the morning huddle, perhaps of a tooth for which we'd previously recommended a full coverage restoration, but upon which the patient has not yet completed treatment. It could be a suspicious soft-tissue lesion, a periodontal problem, a fractured filling Melissa has noted, or any number of things we desire both patient and dentist to be allowed to view more clearly, and of which we may desire to capture a more permanent record.

Having any of the previously described situations on screen when I arrive helps educate the patient, alerts or reminds me of a concern, and saves me having to wait, or return to discuss things with the patient a second time, after the image is taken. Such forced return visits are avoidable delays that, when repeated several times a day, drive me nuts! (Yes, it well may be more of a putt than a drive, in my case.)

If the dentist has still not arrived when the hygiene assistant's tasks are completed, she returns to the intercom to announce, "Doctor, Mr. Businessman is ready in Room 1 for his **second check**." This is the dentist's notification that it's now past time to perform this examination. (Don't you wish you always had two chances to get things right?)

This period, between first and second check notifications, is the 20-minute window of examination opportunity I mentioned previously. It is of great help to me to be able to time my hygiene patient examination so it interferes as little as possible with other patients' care.

Often, I will have completed my current patient's treatment before the second call from hygiene, and be able to do the recare exam without anyone waiting. Sometimes, I can administer anesthesia to my next patient, then excuse myself to do the exam while the local takes effect. At the very least, I can plan an optimal time to interrupt care during a long case, and tell the patient, "You're doing great! You deserve a break!" Nobody's very disappointed to be allowed to close their mouth and relax, maybe use the rest room, or just stand and stretch for a few minutes. This is especially true if such an interlude is couched as a well-deserved reward for great patient behavior!

Having two rooms available for strictly hygiene use means NEVER HAVING TO DELAY THE EXPENSIVE TALENT THAT IS THE HYGIENIST BY REQUIRING HIM OR HER TO WAIT FOR THE DENTIST TO SHOW UP TO COMPLETE THE EXAMINATION. It also means never forcing the hygienist to interrupt care to allow the dentist's exam, resulting in the hygienist's running behind schedule.

Employing this system, I almost always do exams on already clean mouths, which makes diagnosis easier. The hygiene assistant is totally interruptible, usually having plenty of time to perform her assigned tasks, so I do the exam at any time after her "first check" call.

The hygiene assistant charts and takes notes during the dentist's examination, allowing the hygienist to continue the clinical care for which he or she is highly compensated and uniquely qualified, in the tranquility of the adjacent room. Reflect on the daily expense you fritter away while the hygienist charts for your examination, or listens to you talk golf with your patients seven or eight times a day! (Only Divine Intervention can save our schedule when a fellow hunter is in the office!) While hard to precisely quantify, I'm certain such wasted hygiene salary represents a significant amount of lost dollars over the course of one's career.

The examination completed, the assistant appoints the patient for his next recare visit (on one of our five treatment room computers), prints out insurance papers on the computer, and escorts him to the front office. She then returns to the operatory, sterilizes instruments and prepares the room for the following patient.

When the assistant hears the hygienist begin to depart from her patient, she seats the next patient in the already prepared room, then goes next door to complete care on the patient the hygienist has just finished treating. This pattern is repeated--efficiently and profitably-throughout the day.

In-Room Hygiene Scheduling

I'd strongly suggest hygiene personnel schedule recare themselves, as fewer people involved in any system decrease the chances of errors occurring. (When hygiene appoints in the operatory, there is no chance a failed communication with the front office could lead to some embarrassing error in scheduling.)

No one knows more accurately than the person who has just completed care how the next appointment should ideally be scheduled. The hygienist can allocate the preferred interval between visits--this could be anywhere from two to 12 months--in our practice. She can request precisely the time needed for the treatment of every unique patient, based on a history of anxiety, plaque and tartar build-up, root sensitivity, etc. This time can include 10 minutes to chat with Ms. Lonely, if one accepts the inevitable fate that one indeed will be chatting, whether the time is available or not.

Also, if the hygienist is paid on commission--a suggestion I highly recommend, and will more fully elucidate in a moment--his or her compensation will depend on each patient's understanding and committing to diagnosed and recommended periodontal treatment. This fiscal reality enhances the tendency for the advantages of preventive care to be fully addressed and stressed by the hygiene team with every patient, as the hygienist's salary is directly affected by his or her ability to gain patient treatment acceptance. (Just as it is for us dentists.)

Hygienist Compensation

On the **FIRST DAY** our office switched to compensation based on percentage of production--I'd estimate this fortuitous event occurred about 12 years ago--our hygiene revenue **increased 25 percent** and has never retreated from this elevated status. (Please note my emphasis on the **FIRST** day. It did not take months for my hygienist to grasp, then take wholesome advantage of her opportunity to significantly enhance her income by offering care more effectively! Her daddy raised no fools!)

One can argue it is an employee's duty to work as hard as possible, regardless of the level of compensation. Right! The Soviet Union vigorously examined this philosophy of labor without chance of enhanced personal gain, without notable success. It's a simple fact: Most people will gladly work harder if given an opportunity to make more money for a greater effort.

Assume you saw a long-time patient for an emergency visit at day's end, Doctor. The front office had advised you she'd fractured the lingual cusp off #5. A PAX had already been taken by your outstanding chairside. You've done multiple crowns on this well-paying patient. There are no insurance concerns. Under such circumstances, I was always happy to stay late and perform the crown prep immediately.

Treating one additional patient wasn't a big deal, and this represents a nice boost to the day's production. One staff member would volunteer to work late--overhead for this procedure would be minimal--and the loyal patient was grateful for the prompt attention.

(I always ASK a staff member to stay in situations where definitive treatment is an option I chose. Dental team members well understand their obligation to work until all scheduled and true emergency care is completed, but in cases such as I've described above, the level of care offered is based on my whim, and staff have lives and evening plans too. Under these circumstances, it's merely polite to request a volunteer. I can't recall a single time one of my dedicated team wasn't willing to stay. But realize the dentist is adding at least $600 to production. The assistant's incentive to work late is considerably less motivating.)

There's no way in the world I'd have done the prep that evening if I were on a fixed salary. How about you? (I spent two years in the Army Dental Corps, so I know this is true for me.)

Another advantage of compensation by percentage of production: It used to bug me to see my highly reimbursed hygienist enjoying a cup of coffee during "open time," still receiving her hourly salary. When earnings are based on production, I'm happy to provide the coffee, but I'm not paying for her time as she sips.

I've heard concerns that a hygienist won't perform his or her job as thoroughly-will rush, miss areas of debris, cause patients pain-if compensated by percentage. If the dentist checks each patient, as required by law, he or she should note any remaining areas of calculus. A skilled and dedicated staff should hear and repeat any complaints of roughness, even if the dentist is not directly informed by patients.

These concerns should not present a problem. In fact, quality of care should increase when hygiene compensation is tied to productivity. I believe hygienists will understand that doing everything within their power to promote the office and establish long-term, positive patient relationships is in their best interests, as they won't be paid to treat patients who don't return for treatment.

I can only speak from personal experience, but in all candor, I've employed associate dentists who were deficient in skill and/or motivation, and whose work has been suspect. (Come to think of it, my stuff has been "iffy" at times.) Despite some minor interpersonal problems with one past hygienist, I have never experienced a lack of professionalism, skill or dedication from any hygienist within my office over the 26 years I've employed them.

Why go to all this bother? Two rooms and a full-time assistant dedicated to hygiene? While many intangibles can be identified in favor of the system--such as the psychological advantages of establishing a supportive hygiene team to help stave off the hungry wolf of emotional rejection that might tempt your hygienist to explore other practice opportunities--the definitive answer lies in an analysis of the numbers. **(It's about PROFIT, remember?)**

Our Office Numbers from Expanded Hygiene

I am going to illustrate my proposal, using data from my office, where, as I've mentioned, we have collectively reaped the fruits of expanded hygiene for approximately 15 years. Please digest the concepts and hard numbers illustrated here, then employ fee and salary figures from your own office to personalize and enhance the meaning of my example.

Some of you may be concerned that my results won't be representative of your situation. True, Keokuk, Iowa, IS the Mecca of fine dentistry. But remember, I am one of nine dentists practicing in a

Midwestern community of 13,000--mostly blue-collar--souls. I'm not good-looking, charming, sophisticated, or particularly pleasant-smelling...although I do have my own teeth!

Insurance fees are low for our rural area, significantly below those paid in the Iowa City, Iowa, area (a community 95 miles due north of Keokuk), where the level of dental excellence is seemingly perceived to be notably better by omniscient insurers, and/or providing care deemed much more expensive. (I'll list all our periodontal fees later.)

I have employed four hygienists during our 15 years of expanded hygiene, and have had similar fiscal results with each. Five associates have provided the great majority of the examination support for hygiene over that period. (Some years my effort devoted to patient care occurred as infrequently as three days per month. Yes, I meant month.)

In short, it's sure as hell not me, it's not the practice, it's not the community, it's not the hygienist, ancillary staff or dentist...it's the system that creates the amazing results we are about to examine. And any office that chooses to emulate our system can create similar results.

When we began utilizing two rooms and a dedicated hygiene assistant, we were instantly able to expand our scheduled hygiene patients from eight to 12 a day. (Not bad, an instant 50 percent increase in production.)

In the pre-expanded era, our hygienist spent roughly an hour with each patient. Today, with two staff seeing an average of 12 patients daily, each client receives an average of 80 minutes of staff time. (Sixteen total hours of care--eight hours from two staff members--divided among 12 patients = (16 / 12 = 1 1/3 hours per patient.) This extra attention leads to enhanced educational opportunities, more effective relationship building, and a resultant increase in case acceptance, plus augmented number and quality of referrals. ("At my dentist's office, they take their time, I never feel rushed, and they always answer all my questions!")

As the astute may recall from the introduction, during 1999, Melissa produced an average of $133 per hour. Thus a single hygienist, working an eight-hour day, generated a daily production of (8 x $133) = $1,064. If patients were seen a conservative 200 days annually, total hygiene production would be (200 x $1,064) = $212,800.

Our actual 1999 totals were 163 eight-hour days of hygiene worked and $173,270 produced. This diminished total of days and dollars was partially the result of no associates being employed. I worked a four-day week--that seemed like eight--and took some vacation time, when the entire office was closed.

(It had been many years since our office had been closed, even for summer vacation. I'd forgotten what it felt like to work hard for three weeks, take one week off, and forfeit 50 percent of one's monthly net. Just so we're clear, to me, it didn't feel good!)

Closing the office for these days (200 - 163 = 37 lost days) cost me, in lost hygiene production alone, ($212,800 - $173,270 =) $39,530. Since much of our fixed overhead is already paid, the majority of this production is lost NET. (Grant me a moment to regain my composure. Lost profit touches me deeply!)

Take a moment and focus on our actual 1999 hygiene production total of $173,270. Chances are you saw patients for more than our 163 days a year. Use our average production of $1,064 per day to consider how our results compare to your current hygiene production. It will also prove enlightening to compare our results to published national standards.

According to the May 1998 *Dental Economics* practice survey article, the average hygienist produced $6,835 per month or $82,000 per year. *Dental Economics* didn't break these numbers down any further, but if we assume a 40-hour week, this calculates out to $43 per hour. Melissa produced at a rate approximately TRIPLE this hourly level! ($133 / $43 = 3).

I hope each reader is motivated by the realization that if such production is achieved in our little country office, it is possible in his or her office also, even if one practices in such backwaters as New York City or San Francisco.

Sure be nice if you got to keep all that money! You don't, so let's examine overhead. (My focus on NET never wavers.) Your hygienist will probably wish to be paid. (Most seem to.) Let's assume one is at least considering my suggestion to establish hygiene compensation based on a percentage of production. The harder one's hygienist chooses to work, the greater her compensation...just like you, doctor.

Depending on the availability of hygienists in one's practice area (the law of supply and demand has not been repealed!), let's forecast a range of remuneration from 20% ($26.60 per hour at $133 production) to 33 percent ($43.89 per hour at $133 production).

To enhance these figures' relevance with some local data, our wonderfully talented Melissa, with six years of previous experience, was being paid $14.50 per hour by a nearby practice, from which we rescued her.

Hygiene assistant is an entry-level position in our office, requiring outstanding people skills more than dental experience and expertise. (We'll detail the hygiene assistant's duties shortly.) Let's assume the beginning salary range for this team member varies from $7 to $10 per hour, the difference primarily based on average pay in one's geographic area.

(I realize practitioners on either coast, or in major metropolitan areas, may have to multiply my overhead numbers by two or three to make them applicable to their situation. I can only relate what has been my experience, and do so while thanking God I practiced in an area where overhead and living expenses are relatively modest.)

One must factor in overhead in addition to salary--a difficult figure to precisely define for hygiene--but in our low-overhead, highly efficient office (our practice averaged 48 percent overhead during the last three years that I worked with associates), this totals approximately $18 per hour of hygiene care.

This $18 overhead beyond salary is my best educated guess. I arrived at this figure by noting that hygiene produced about 25 percent of our total office revenue. (The commonly quoted ideal for hygiene production is 33 percent of the office total, but poor Melissa had to compete with up to three dentists.) I assumed 25 percent of rent, phone, utilities and front-office salary was dedicated to hygiene's behalf.

I had a staff member total typical hygiene supply expenses (gloves, prophy paste, disposable prophy heads, fluoride, toothbrushes, floss, etc.) for a six-month period, and doubled this figure to estimate annual total dollars of hygiene supply expenses. Adding all the above-listed items results in total hygiene non-salary expenses. I divided this figure by the number of hours hygiene saw patients during the year reviewed (this figure recorded on the practice monitors we'll soon examine) to reach this $18 hourly estimate. Again, this is merely my best educated guess.

We have now established a low range of $26.60 (hygienist's salary) plus $7 (assistant salary) plus $18 (non-salary overhead), or $51.60 per hour of total overhead, to a high range of $43.89 plus $10 plus $18, or $71.89 per hour of total overhead. **At $133-per-hour production, this leaves the practice with a remaining hygiene prof-**

it of from $61.11 to $81.40 per hour. ($133 - $51.60 = $81.40. $133 - $71.89 = $61.11.)

(Recall the *Dental Economics* figure for average hygiene production--not net profit--was $43 per hour.) Based on 200 eight-hour days, we're discussing an **annual NET PROFIT ranging from (200 days x 8 hours x $61.11 net/hour = $98,000) to (200 days x 8 hours x $81.40 net/hour = $130,240) occurring from hygiene alone!**

Melissa is paid 20.1% of production. (I'll describe how we arrived at this somewhat unusual figure later.) Her assistant's salary is $8 per hour, so our office net figures are almost at the highest end of our profitability scale of $81.40 per hour. For 163 days worked, at $81.40 net per hour, my best possible guesstimate of our actual hygiene net profit was **$106,500** for 1999. ($81.40 per hour x 8 hours x 163 days = $106,500.)

If this illustration of $98,000 to $130,240 profit from hygiene production alone has failed to excite you, take a pulse! Many dentists-I assume those too busy to bother with system refinement-struggle to reach such profit totals for their entire office!

One personalizes this data by repeating my overhead computations with figures from his or her practice to determine:

a) one's profit or loss from current hygiene.
b) the potential that exists with expanded hygiene.

(Remember that all hygiene overhead except a few additional supplies, added assistant salary, and a well-earned increase in hygienist's compensation is fixed, so **the additional 50 percent production, which is virtually assured by going from eight to 12 patients treated per day, is mostly net profit!)**

The above calculations are all one needs to determine the current profitability of one's hygiene department...if one has the stones to look! (Recall the motto of the unsuccessful dentists: God save us from the truth!)

Hypothetical Calculations

I'm about to indulge in a pastime that, at least while writing about dental matters, I attempt strictly to avoid: **I'm going to make something up!** Please understand this is a hypothetical example, useful only to illustrate a bare-bones comparison between conventional and expanded hygiene, the numbers included being nothing more than experienced conjecture on my part.

Let's consider a hygiene department that treats an average of seven patients a day for a prophy fee of $49, resulting in $343 per-day production--very close to the *Dental Economics* $344 per-day average. (I hope every dentist employing a hygienist would AT LEAST KNOW THE AVERAGE DAILY PRODUCTION OF THIS DEPARTMENT. If you don't know, find out, but please calculate your accurate net profit from hygiene by entering your actual practice's figures into my calculations.)

I'm using a seven-patient average to take into consideration the failed appointments, unfilled cancellations and just plain unscheduled open time that unavoidably appear on most hygiene schedules. (But, as we'll observe when we consider hygiene monitors in a later chapter, rarely on our schedule.)

Let's **make up** a hygienist's salary of $20 per hour, for a total gross salary of $160 per eight-hour day. (This is NOT a suggested compensation--plenty of people are already mad at me--merely a very **MODEST** estimate.) Add to this a non-salary expense of $12 per hour (**made up**), times eight hours = $96 per day. (I generously assumed other overhead will be reduced by one third from our $18 figure, as without expanded hygiene, one treats one third less patients. However, I know, due to predominantly fixed costs--rent, utilities, salary--actual savings will be less than this.)

Thus we have total non-expanded daily hygiene overhead of $160 salary + $96 non-salary = $256. Reducing our $343 of production by this amount leaves a total of ($343 - $256 =) $87 net profit per day. **Compare this to our expanded hygiene NET of $61.11 to $81.40 PER HOUR!**

And this illustration is with a MINIMAL $20 hygienist salary. Net decreases from this total by the amount salary exceeds $20. (Could you place an MO composite during the time it takes to conduct seven examinations? What about two units of crown and bridge preparation at $1,200? Is the frustration level of fiscally aware dentists with their hygiene departments' low profitability now easier to understand? But don't blame hygienists if the practice owner hasn't devised and implemented a system that maximizes profit potential.)

These rough (**made-up**) calculations are in no way inclusive, as they make no attempt to consider x-rays, sealants, etc. on the revenue side; or Social Security, Medicare, workmen's compensation, and the inevitable five-patient day (when $245 production results in a negative $11 net) as overhead considerations.

When my thought processes (using **made-up data**) are supplemented by accurate figures from your office, I hope these scribbles--their meaning enhanced by comparison to my office's actual expanded hygiene figures--will allow additional light to be shed on the extraordinary profit potential of expanded hygiene.

One's calculations should clearly illustrate that adding a hygiene assistant will present no financial burden. Can one justify adding a room of equipment to make this concept feasible? If one has the additional space, the practice should be able to pay for top-of-the-line equipment from increased hygiene production alone in about six weeks. Even at our most conservative annual figure of $98,000, one can finance the building or expansion of an office easily on expanded hygiene NET alone.

One last critical hurdle exists: Do you have the patient load to keep an expanded hygiene schedule productive? Even if one's current hygienist is completely booked, a 50 percent increase in patient load (from eight to 12 daily patients) is required to make the system viable.

This isn't a decision one reaches emotionally, but analytically. Twelve patients a day x 200 days = 2,400 annual patient visits. A well-run office with 1,200 active patients should be able to fill this time, as no consideration for new patient care, sealant placement, and multiple visit soft-tissue therapy is included.

To determine your practice's active patient count, select one foot of files at random, and count the number of patients within that segment of files that have been seen in one's office over the last 18 months. (You'll have to look inside each file to determine date last seen.)

Now measure the total length of all files, and multiply the number of active patients counted in the examined one-foot section times total feet of files that exist to determine active patient count (i.e., 50 active patients in the one foot of files audited, times 40 feet of total files = 2,000 active patients).

To aid those with fewer than 1,200 patients, I will advance multiple suggestions to enhance one's level of patient flow--all ideas which our office has successfully implemented for years--in a following segment.

But Where Do I Go from Here?

Begin by sharing this information with one's hygienist. Don't be reluctant to reveal my projections of enhanced office net. Our professions must enter an era where dentists and hygienists understand their compensation depends on MUTUAL SUCCESS and teamwork. Your hygienist should be more interested in his or her new salary estimates than in your potential profits.

Before approaching your hygienist, be certain you have completed your homework by using office fees and production figures from YOUR practice, to make the example personally and profoundly relevant. (This simple preparation is something any businessperson would routinely perform before advancing a proposal. If you wish to be compensated as a businessperson, **act like one!**) Dentistry may be the only industry embarrassed or reluctant to create a system that improves staff compensation, enhances patient care AND increases the owner's net--an example of the free-enterprise system performing at its finest.

(Considering our profession's dearth of formal business training, and the resultant modest level of the average dentist's business acumen, it's no wonder third parties threaten to engulf our profession. Every motivated reader of this book should become skilled well beyond the average practitioner in business understanding, if they do no more than carefully evaluate the profitability of their hygiene department!)

Success with expanded hygiene requires the complete and enthusiastic cooperation of one's hygienist. I strongly suggest enlisting his or her zealous support for these proposed practice improvements, by offering to change compensation from hourly or straight weekly or monthly salary, to a percentage of production.

To reach an equitable salary percentage for one's office, take total hygiene production from the last calendar year, and divide that into the hygienist's total W-2 compensation for that year.

If the income figure was $28,600, and production was $100,000, one's new agreement would establish his or her hygienist's salary at ($28,600 salary / $100,000 production =) 28.6 percent of production.

If production for the following year was again $100,000, the hygienist's compensation, though now determined as a percentage of production, would be unchanged. But, for every dollar above $100,000 produced, the hygienist would earn an additional 28.6 cents. (Again, 28.6 percent is not a suggested compensation, merely an example to illustrate how easily and accurately percentage of hygiene production paid in salary can be calculated...especially if production is an even $100,000! It is a one-step, one-time division problem...but I went to dental school too. If you aren't sure you've got it right, have your accountant double-check.)

What about paid benefits? All benefits from the preceding year are already included in the hygienist's W-2 information, so every existing perquisite--paid vacation, holidays, sick leave, continuing education, paid staff meeting time, prophys for fellow staff, family and perhaps friends of the practice, for which there was no charge, but for which a salary was paid--are already contained within our hypothetical 28.6 percent.

Be very clear here. While there is no longer a need for separate accounting of benefits, these fringe-benefit dollars haven't been eliminated, but are already **automatically factored into the total compensation package.**

It has been my experience that hygienists are hard-working professionals, as enthusiastic about enhancing performance and income as any dentist. The idea of two rooms, plus their own assistant dedicated to hygiene, should be attractive--perceived as the ideal working environment--if presented properly. The data we've shared should excite both dentist and hygienist with the vision of a more mutually fulfilling and financially rewarding future.

I'd never hesitate to guarantee a minimum salary equal to what the hygienist was receiving before modifications to expanded hygiene began, and compensation changed to percentage of production. Assuming your staff has the ability to fill the schedule, there seems no possible way, while seeing 12 patients a day, one could produce less than he or she had when seeing eight patients a day.

Let me confuse you in the name of clarity. (Who said I've been doing that for many pages?) Our office has always included dentist examinations as a portion of hygiene production. We've done this as, when we first converted to hygiene compensation based on percentage of production, our past records included examinations as part of hygiene production.

These old figures had no influence on compensation--we then paid our hygienist an hourly salary--but were compiled only to help us monitor our hygiene department's progress. To establish a compensation percentage, we had to either go back and remove all examinations done during the previous year (this was B.C.--before computers), or leave examinations in our production total. It should come as no surprise to attentive readers that I chose the easiest way.

This concept seems to perplex folks, but when determining the percentage of production to be paid as hygiene compensation, it makes no difference in final salary paid if examinations are left in or removed. Calculated either way--with or without examinations--the forthcoming percentage assures identical production will result in identical future compensation. The percent figure will change, based on excluding or including exams, but the final dollar compensation paid for identical treatment won't be altered.

Assume $100 in production, that included an examination, times an agreed-upon 25 percent compensation = $25 hygiene salary. The same patient will create $80 in hygiene production, when a $20 examination fee is removed. The hygiene compensation has been adjusted up to 32 percent (to reflect exam production lost), so hygiene salary would now be $80 x 32 percent = $25. The change in production is balanced by the adjustment in compensation, so equal work still receives equal pay.

Of course, hygienists aren't allowed to perform examinations by law, and if one can easily remove exam fees from hygiene production figures, this would be ideal. But to me, the added clarity hardly seemed worth forcing someone to re-figure a year of data to accomplish this objective.

Hygienists sometimes fear expanded hygiene will leave them burned-out "scaling machines." Just the opposite is true. Freed of the drudgery--unless he or she enjoys exposing and developing x-rays, scrubbing instruments, reviewing medical histories, cleaning and setting up rooms, giving oral hygiene instructions, etc.--the work environment becomes more pleasant while it grows more productive.

Allow me to present the definitive example of this contention for any dentist to comprehend: Would you enjoy working a day without a chairside? I admit to being spoiled by my wonderful staff, but if I were forced to work without an assistant, I'd reschedule the day without a second thought.

Expanded hygiene allows patients to experience more individual staff time and attention (80 minutes versus 60 minutes), thus improving dental education, further cementing office bonds, enhancing the overall dental experience, while stimulating increased case acceptance and enhanced quality and quantity of referrals.

If widely adopted, expanded hygiene would end the national shortage of licensed hygienists, as employing our system means each dental office not currently practicing in an expanded mode is now capable of an instant 50 percent increase in patient care.

As our illustration of accelerated hourly net unquestionably demonstrates, it is much more profitable and efficient for even an office that currently has patient demand below the level required to schedule full-time hygiene to implement part-time expanded hygiene, say two days a week, instead of regular, less profitable hygiene three or four days a week.

Rather than injuring the hygiene profession, expansion allows increased remuneration--**without decreasing owner's net**--plus improved hygienists' working conditions, as tedious jobs are shifted to less skilled staff.

In most practices, if one's hygienist requests a raise, without advancing a plan to increase his or her productive capabilities, said salary increase, if granted, must be paid by decreasing the dentist's profit. (The pie didn't become larger, it's just sliced differently.) As a hard-working dentist, toiling to the same degree for less recompense is not a thought upon which I like to dwell. If such a salary request is granted, the dentist might be resentful. If refused, the hygienist might be exploring employment opportunities. Expanded hygiene is the only plan of which I'm aware that allows everyone to win.

As we've clearly seen, this markedly more profitable expanded hygiene department creates extraordinary higher net for the office from hygiene production alone. In addition, performing 12 daily exams, rather than the previous eight, will lead to diagnosis of additional restorative needs, and thus increase demand for the dentist's services, especially if the hygiene assistant uses the intra-oral camera as effectively as we've previously described.

Our office insists every tooth we crown have a PAX and intra-oral photo taken before treatment is begun. Sending the photo, along with a properly completed form, greatly facilitates dealing with insurance queries--in fact, my front office staff claims that including photos almost eliminates questions concerning coverage for fixed restorations.

We also take photos before, during and after periodontal treatment. This is helpful with insurance, and for legal documentation, but most importantly, allowing the patient to observe the condition of the teeth and tissues so clearly--and almost all periodontal patients are SHOCKED by a magnified look at the lingual of the mandibular anteriors--is a great motivator. When one mandibular quadrant has been treated, the other not, a view of the difference in appearance between healing and unhealthy tissue is highly educational and motivational for the patient undergoing care.

In summary, expanded hygiene is the gas pedal for overall office acceleration. What knowledgeable dentist wouldn't be supportive and committed to nurturing a profit center of this magnitude?

Now let's consider more specific treatment concerns, including fee and insurance information.

Chapter 3

Soft Tissue Procedures and Fees

Before we proceed with a discussion of procedures, fees and insurance data, let me suggest that if one is serious about maximizing hygiene, it is incumbent upon the dentist and hygienist to hone their expertise concerning soft tissue or periodontal treatment. Allow me to suggest two fine courses that can quickly and inexpensively jump-start one's hygiene department. I've attended both, and found each enjoyable and useful.

Dr. Rick Kushner, of Lean and Mean seminar fame, offers an excellent and pragmatic course on hygiene. Rick is a marvelously successful dentist, who wastes not a word in either lecture or office. He'll provide the red meat, all the vital factual knowledge one needs to jump into expanded hygiene on the run. One may obtain information concerning all of Rick's extraordinarily useful products and activities by calling 1-303-277-0001.

I understand Rick has decided to cut down on the number of speaking engagements he accepts. Nobody can understand this more than I, who retired to do whatever I damn well wish at age 53. I'm a firm believer in the wisdom of personal freedom, the essential ingredient of creativity. (Really hard work--including lots of THINKING!!-is a close second.) But losing Rick's talents as a speaker is a catastrophe for dentistry. This guy is unique! If there has been, in the history of the universe, a more innovative and financially successful dentist than Rick, I haven't heard of him or her!

Pro-Dentec®, manufacturer of the Rota-dent toothbrush our office has incorporated in our soft tissue treatment system for many years, also offers superb courses. (Pro-Dentec coined the now ubiquitous phrase, Soft Tissue Management.) As an added value, I purchased the two piezo scalers Melissa and her patients love from these nice folks--at a significant discount--while attending their program.

I'm not an easy guy to please--ask anyone--but the Pro-Dentec staff I've come to know over the years are exceptional people, enthusiastic about their services, products and jobs, and always willing to go the extra mile to accommodate their clients.

I'm no expert on electric brushes, although I'd estimate I've ordered and personally tried around 15 brands. My personal preference--and what I've seen work best for our patients--is Rota-dent. When patients faithfully comply with our recommendations regarding Rota-dent use, all involved are pleased by the wonderful tissue improvement we invariably observe. Also, the company has never disappointed our office concerning service or support for any of their products. (Life is too short to deal with people one can't trust or depend on.) Pro-Dentec may be reached by calling 1-800-228-5595.

I'm sure many other fine periodontal courses are available, but these are the two from which I've benefited the most. Both unerringly focus, not on the biology of the inflammatory reaction, the complexity of various micro-surgery procedures, or other such fascinating (but to me USELESS) minutiae, but on precisely how to establish an efficient, profitable hygiene department that offers state-of-the-art soft tissue care.

In the nature of full disclosure, allow me to share our hygiene fees, not to suggest what another office should charge--as every practice situation is unique, and fees must reflect this--but to enhance meaning when one compares his or her hygiene production numbers to ours.

(An area that can charge $70 for a routine cleaning varies significantly, at least in a business sense, from one where the typical fee is $40. To put our practice results-detailed in the preceding chapter-into proper perspective requires that one clearly understands how our charges relate to the fees in your area and office.)

We offer five levels of soft tissue management, the degree of individual care required determined by the periodontal status of the patient. I won't get into precise clinical descriptions--the class of cleaning is based upon the periodontal charting Melissa and her assistant perform, and details are best left to the experts like Dr. Kushner and the fine folks at Pro-Dentec to detail--but here are our five prophy levels, complete with fees, the ADA codes our office files, and ROUGH description.

(These fees were as of 1 January, 2000. I'd suggest an annual increase of about 4 percent per year. Such an adjustment will make the data meaningful, whenever one peruses this text. Thus a $50 fee one year later--January, 2001--would be adjusted by $50 x 4% = $2, or $52.)

Class A. This is a basic cleaning of stain and light super-gingival tartar, with little or no inflammation present, for which we charge $51. We bill these procedures under ADA code 1110.

Class B. This is a heavier prophy, frequently required after a patient is past due for his or her routine cleaning. While stain and debris may be heavy, there should be little inflammation, bleeding or pocketing. Our fee is $86. We also bill these under ADA code 1110.

If one charges a standard Class A fee for a prophy that is provided months past the professionally recommended interval of periodontal maintenance, the unmistakable message given to the patient is that the cleaning is unimportant, and the dentist and/or hygienist-suggested time intervals are insignificant or contrived.

Such an unintended but obvious message is unfair to one's office, to the hygienist who must provide care--often made much more difficult due to the delay, and with insufficient time now available--and **not consistent with maintaining ideal oral health for one's patients. IT IS NEVER ACCEPTABLE--PROFESSIONALLY, MORALLY OR LEGALLY--TO ALLOW LESS THAN OPTIMAL PERIODONTAL HEALTH IN THE PATIENTS WHO TRUST YOU FOR THEIR DENTAL CARE.**

One must explain, in a behaviorally sound fashion, how long after the recommended recall interval the patient has arrived. We don't judge or criticize overdue patients, as doing so makes them reluctant to come back. (Lecturing patients who finally do show up is like beating your hunting dog after he's obeyed your command to "come." No matter what either has done, the message ingested by the dog and patient is not to show up again.)

I often tell them, "I'm just glad you're here now." But we do carefully demonstrate why additional time and expense will be required to complete their treatment. We also don't hesitate to reappoint a patient to complete overdue care. We advise the patient that we wish to finish the procedure in about two weeks, after allowing some time for HEALING--which is what occurs as DISEASE disappears.

(We DON'T mention that completing his or her care on the spot would also throw our entire day off schedule, making committed people who kept suggested recare intervals wait. Consider that information as our little secret.)

Mirror and/or intra-oral camera must be employed to illustrate problems or areas of concern, thus demonstrating that more frequent cleanings are needed, why a second appointment may be required, and why the fee must be increased. To do less--perhaps not being completely candid due to a lack of total commitment, or fear of rejection-is to fail in one's professional duty to obtain and maintain the patient's ideal oral health.

Let's get this critical point straight. It is our duty, as healthcare professionals, to advise patients what and when care is needed. If they choose not to follow our advice, and problems result, our obligation includes pointing out this reality--in a helpful and non-judgmental manner--and clearly describing what must occur to regain ideal oral health.

As part of the morning huddle we discussed previously, the number of months any scheduled patient is behind our recommended interval for treatment is noted on the daily schedule, and this data highlighted with yellow. This deficiency will be mentioned at least twice, by dentist and hygienist, during the patient's visit. The critical importance of timely care--thus reducing cost, increasing comfort, requiring fewer appointments and enhancing the level of periodontal health--will be clarified and emphasized.

For any patients with gingival bleeding, recent studies linking periodontal disease to systemic conditions including stroke, cardiovascular disease, ulcers, lung disease, diabetes, low birth weight babies, and other maladies are discussed. Patients are provided with copies of articles from dental journals relating this relationship, and, most impressively to them, a reprint of a *Consumer Reports* article from a couple of years ago discussing periodontal disease and care.

For years our treatment notes repeatedly contained such messages as, "Patient still has some bleeding. Reviewed OH, stressed floss. Apt. 6 mo. recall." A WATERSHED MOMENT in the history of our office occurred when we, as a team, committed to no longer accepting **active bacterial infection**--that's what makes gums bleed, and is always the phrase I use to describe it to achieve maximum impact--as allowable. We vowed to offer whatever care was required to stop this disease process for every patient. The information relating bleeding gums to systemic health was developed years later, and only served to strengthen our commitment and resolve.

We do, however, in the holy name of sanity, follow the precepts of the **Singing Pig Rule.** This states, "Don't try to teach pigs to sing. It wastes your time, and it annoys the pigs." We understand there exist finite limits to anyone's ability to motivate others to change behavior. We don't waste time giving "singing lessons" to people who clearly don't care.

Class C. This is a quagmire. Not frank disease, but an unsightly mess, with heavy stain and calculus accumulations, but without significant pocketing or bone loss.

Any patient with suspected class C or ABOVE cleaning is scheduled for full-mouth periodontal charting--billed under ADA code 4110, our fee being $52. I spot-probe every new patient, but under conditions such as seen with class C cases, isolated areas of significant pocketing could be hiding beneath all the debris. A full-mouth probing by our expert, Melissa, is indicated.

Also, I don't want to get in trouble for incorrectly scheduling the required periodontal treatment. If I improperly classify a patient (as C, D, or F), insufficient time may be available to complete his or her care, as well as an insufficient fee being paid for the level of care delivered. Hygienists paid on commission aren't too pleased about either of these inadequacies! Our fee for a class C prophy is $119 plus $52 for charting, for a total of $171. We bill this under ADA code 4345.

Class D. Make no mistake, this level of care and beyond are periodontal treatments--not a cleaning. Multiple pockets, many in the 5 mm or greater range, will be present, most with bleeding. Anesthetic will be used, and the entire treatment process will include three visits-two for 1/2-mouth scalings, and a third regular prophy and healing check. Our fee is $52 for charting, $96 per quadrant plus $51 for the final prophy appointment--a total of $487. We bill this under ADA code 4341.

(The great solons from the state of Iowa began allowing hygienists to administer local anesthesia about two years ago. Melissa took the required course, and having her administer anesthesia as needed for periodontal patients has been a great aid to me. No more coming into a room, saying hello to a trembling patient, then giving eight injections and leaving. Such is the level of Melissa's talents that she's never once required me to help her achieve profound anesthesia. Tempting as it's been, I'm too proud--or too insecure--to request Melissa to help me get some recalcitrant patient numb.)

Class F. This is a D gone sour. Lots of 7 mm or greater pockets, with heavy bleeding and often suppuration. Treatment will be completed using anesthesia and be spread over five appointments. (One quadrant per visit, plus a regular prophy and healing check at the end of care.) Our fee for charting is $52, plus $161 per quadrant and $51 for the final visit for a total investment of $747. (This fee has a slightly mystical aspect, as these folks have pockets within which one could hide a small Boeing aircraft.)

A Rota-dent toothbrush is automatically added to all C, D and F treatments. We also suggest a Rota-dent to any patient with a history of periodontal disease, or any current bleeding, no matter what point in our A to F universe we happen to stumble upon them. We charge a fee of $126 per brush, and bill it under ADA code 4342. Many dentists choose to lump the brush in with total treatment fee. We have always billed it separately, for two reasons.

1. I wish every patient to know this is a costly and sophisticated dental device...not just another toothbrush. Being aware of the INVESTMENT required increases patients' understanding of our desired goal of involving this instrument in the regular, effective removal of oral bacteria several times a day.
2. For some patients, the brush must be broken out to gain maximum possible insurance benefits. Had we not revealed the level of investment required beforehand, we'd risk losing the patients' trust if they felt we were trying to "sneak" this expensive instrument in without them being aware of the cost.

The advantage for NOT separating the brush fee from total treatment investment is avoiding arguments about accepting this instrument. I feel explaining the Rota-dent's importance to be part of our educational mission. I also understand why some offices would choose to lump the cost with overall treatment. How this is best handled is a judgment call, but I've discovered, through numerous painful and discouraging experiences, that patients who refuse to purchase an ideal electric brush seldom complete care.

Every periodontal patient must be made completely aware of the vital role his or her daily cleaning efforts will play in the chances of healing, and remaining free of gum disease. I believe failure to accept the Rota-dent indicates a reluctance to assume such responsibility for one's oral health.

All dentists are aware that, without patient compliance concerning recare and home care, no periodontal treatment can be successful. If a patient is not committed to restoring his or her mouth to optimal health, it saves my stomach lining to discover that unfortunate fact early in our relationship. Failure to invest in a quality home care device often reveals this fact.

Rota-dent sells a single brush to dentists for $69.50. If one orders 12, an extra brush is added free of charge. If one attends Pro-Dentec's seminars, additional discounted specials are offered. We earn our profit by stocking the item, demonstrating and encouraging its use, and standing behind it if repair or replacement is indicated.

Only the very brave or very foolish believe they can solve every problem themselves. (I'm not sure a difference exists between the above-named two parties, so I may need to beg your pardon for my redundancy!) Melissa and the treating dentist (myself or associate) decide when to refer a patient to a periodontist based on disease level, oral hygiene, history of tobacco and/or alcohol abuse, the state of his or her general health, pocket and bleeding information, past compliance record, the mental attitude or temperament of the patient (bitchy or nice), etc.

The skill level of the person providing periodontal therapy should also determine which cases one attempts to treat. Only Melissa offers periodontal therapy in our practice. She is highly skilled, but we still don't try to treat everyone. Basically, we try to transfer cases we fear might fail.

When to refer to a specialist is a personal decision, and I'd rather over-refer than under-refer. But, due to the level of Melissa's ability, our referrals to a periodontist's office are rare. While we suffer our disappointments, I have no recollection of any periodontal patient we've treated ever losing all of his or her teeth.

After initial care is completed, class C, D and F patients are customarily scheduled at three-month intervals for routine recare prophys. Many of these folks stay on three-month intervals forever, which is a powerful motivation to be certain one likes the periodontal patients one chooses to treat. (For the curious, I have no idea what unhappy fate befell the letter E. Perhaps E is considered bad luck, like having a 13th floor in hotels?)

One can't perform periodontal treatment without anesthesia, at prophy fees, during the course of a one-hour appointment, any more than I can do an excellent crown preparation in the time reserved for a class one restoration. Being repeatedly asked to perform such impossible feats of legerdemain, by patients and dentists, is a topic over which hygienists are rightfully frustrated.

To request that prophys be given in a doomed attempt to treat frank periodontal disease compromises professional values. To do so is ineffective, disingenuous, and stupid! On this issue, hygienists have my complete agreement and support. No dental team member should ever knowingly be placed in situations where time and treatment constraints interfere with one's ability to do one's best for his or her patient. Reflect on how you hate being placed in such a predicament, Doctor.

Dentist, hygienist and staff must become educated as to what comprises optimal periodontal treatment, including the use of the several chemical adjuncts available today (brilliantly discussed by Dr. Bader in a following chapter), when and how to chart pocket depths, ideal frequency of recall interval, and many other topics. **If one doesn't comprehend this basic data, get thee to a course immediately, before attempting to upgrade one's hygiene department.** The old saw is true...one can't sell what he or she doesn't have on the shelf.

Take your hygienist, her assistant and a front-office staff member to the training session with you. The courses I've recommended discuss--along with treatment concepts--ideal hygiene scheduling and the wonderland of periodontally related insurance codes.

The insurance codes and fees I've quoted are just how we do things in our office. Again, I claim no expertise, nor am I making suggestions concerning what is an ideal fee--these vary greatly based on geographic location, office overhead, level of expertise, and many other factors--but I wanted you to know the basic figures from which our final financial results are derived.

I'm really no expert on insurance codes. I claim total and blissful ignorance concerning many subjects, but none more profoundly so than insurance. To add to the confusion, the powers that be in the "wacky" world of insurance occasionally change "the right answers," then sit back and enjoy watching dentists try to figure out the newly appropriate codes. The codes I've listed are what Carol May, my invaluable assistant for over 25 years, told me were correct. It is my impression that Carol knows everything. (At least, that's what Carol's always claimed!) If you don't agree with our codes, call her, or keep using whatever works for you.

Additional Hygiene Procedures

Here is a listing of the primary procedures our hygiene department routinely performs, in addition to the afore-discussed A through

F periodontal treatment. These valuable services enhance the excellent level of care we provide, while significantly increasing office revenue.

We stress in-office fluoride treatments, especially for our younger "Mountain Dew Generation" patients; for mature adults, who grow increasingly prone to root caries; and for patients of every age with any active decay. We bill fluoride treatments under ADA code 1204 and charge $28. Adding 12 fluoride treatments a day enhances revenue by (12 x $28 = $336). If you offer care 200 days a year, that's (200 x $336 = $67,200) annual increase in revenue. The natural water in our predominantly rural area contains about one tenth of the ideal fluoride concentration, so supplementation is often desirable and necessary.

New topical fluorides taste good, work quickly, and systems to deliver them are much easier to handle and less messy than formerly. As our aging population keep their teeth longer, and accept more sophisticated restorative care, I feel the importance of fluoride in the fight against root caries becomes increasingly important.

Nothing saddens me more than witnessing an 80-year-old who has enjoyed good natural teeth throughout his or her lifetime, now on multiple medications and suffering severe xerostomia, needing a lot of difficult and expensive restorative care. My advice is to strengthen those vulnerable root surfaces to the highest degree possible, before trouble arrives.

In addition to in-office fluorides, we dispense or write prescriptions for Prevident 5000 for adult patients with exposed roots, active decay, extensive restorative work, or who are undergoing fixed orthodontic treatment. I've used this fluoride source myself for a decade. It's a pleasant-tasting gel, and I believe, still the best product of its kind extant.

For children over age 5 with active caries, we prescribe Colgate's Point Two (.2) fluoride rinse to be used once per week. Kids under the age of 5 may inadvertently swallow when trying to rinse, and this can cause stomach upset. If a pre-5 child has severe decay, I will ask a parent to apply a few drops of .2 on the toothbrush, ideally just before the child goes to bed.

I strongly suggest each parent select a specific day and time to administer this powerful adjunct, to be sure it's not forgotten. I explain that my kids used .2 just before bed every Sunday night. (We live in the country. Until a few years ago, when our residential area was annexed by the city, then provided water from their reservoir, we had a well and didn't enjoy an optimally fluoridated water supply.)

Selling fluoride supplements is a small revenue source for one's office, but we mainly provide it for patient convenience, and to be sure they get the ideal supplement we recommend. When we provide this product, we also know the patient can begin its use immediately. We are happy to call in a prescription for Prevident or .2 for those who have drug discounts as part of their insurance package. All the pharmacies in our area carry these fine fluoride products.

Our office enthusiastically supports sealant use, and has since 1974. We place sealants on ALL kids' permanent molars, seldom on premolars, and almost never on primary teeth. This pattern of usage reflects nothing more than my personal beliefs concerning in what situations sealants prove most effective. We place them on adult teeth with deep, heavily stained, occlusal pits, as I'd want sealants protecting such an area in my own or a loved one's mouth.

Drying the occlusal surface of a typical molar, then showing the pits on our intra-oral camera, results in almost 100 percent acceptance of recommended sealants. If we suggest sealants for a minor with no guardian present, we send an intra-oral photo of such a molar home for Mom to see. It is sometimes useful to compare the cost, and complexity of treatment involved, between sealant placement and the fabrication of an occlusal composite restoration. Once this is accurately understood, most patients choose to protect caries-prone areas with sealants.

Most of the sealants we provide are placed in hygiene, where having a chairside's assistance is invaluable. Our office policy prohibits ANY care provider from placing a sealant without an assistant, as it is my strong feeling that such a solo effort would result in diminished treatment quality. (I'm certain it would if I were the provider, as the critical task of keeping a 6-year-old's lower molar dry during sealant placement is fairly challenging, even when I have help! I refuse to consider that others might possess superior skills allowing them to perform the job well without assistance!) If the hygiene assistant is occupied, a dentist's chairside or front-office staff member is borrowed to facilitate this procedure. (We take sealants very seriously! I've never regretted a sealant I've placed. However, I've often grieved over a virgin tooth the occlusal surface of which has decayed, and that I must now cut.)

Nitrous oxide is available in all five of our operatories, including the two rooms dedicated to hygiene. Nitrous is a big help during periodontal care and sealant application. Nitrous oxide eliminates gag reflexes and slows down the peripatetic movements of kids' tongues, greatly aiding efforts to keep teeth dry while sealants are being placed. Nitrous is ideal for procedures that might prove slightly uncomfortable, but don't require local anesthetic for most patients.

One of the reasons I disliked performing prophys--my last one occurred circa 1975--was that I never knew when I'd cause some discomfort. (At least with operative procedures, one has a pretty good idea of when it might hurt.) Nitrous relaxes the patient, while significantly elevating his or her pain threshold...ideal for uncomfortable but not truly painful treatment. Nitrous' use makes periodontal care easier for patient and provider.

I'll describe exactly how we employ this invaluable adjunct to care in great detail in a later chapter. I have used ONLY NITROUS (no local anesthetic) to restore primary teeth for 20-some years. I still am forced to inject kids for vital pulpotomies, extractions and operative on permanent teeth, but with the help of nitrous, topical, and what I like to call a glacier-slow and feather-gentle technique, they seldom feel the injection. Nitrous proves helpful for many things, but it is a miracle when it comes to making restorative treatment enjoyable for kids, their often anxious parents, and long-suffering dentists and staff!

I mentioned earlier the extreme value of health-care providers' time, and how, in our office, every possible piece of equipment that can enhance efficiency is provided. Both hygiene operatories have plumbed (not portable) nitrous oxide, an x-ray head, intra-oral camera, computer terminal, virtual reality glasses, high-speed fiber optic handpiece (restorative care can be provided in hygiene, but the handpiece is most often used to smooth a chipped tooth or filling, adjust a partial, polish a stained composite, etc.), piezo and ultrasonic scaler...and I'd gladly add anything else Melissa might desire that would further enhance her ability to provide patient care.

My staff and I are all enthusiastic supporters of tooth lightening procedures. (I had my teeth lightened in the early days of the procedure, when drippy, foamy, unpleasant-tasting solutions had to be worn 18 hours a day. I was desperate for ANYTHING THAT MIGHT IMPROVE MY APPEARANCE. So are most of your adult patients! Let's face it, after "a certain age," that swirled past me many moons ago, most of us need all the help we can get!)

Here is the technique that has become Standard Operating Procedure in our office, and has greatly enhanced the number of whitening cases we deliver. Our hygiene assistant asks every patient if he or she is interested in whiter teeth. If the patient responds positively, the assistant immediately takes a shade reading of the upper incisors, and records this data, along with a note on our doctor communication pad requesting the dentist discuss tooth lightening with this patient.

By asking every person we treat, at every visit, we invariably inquire multiple times about any given patient's desire for whiter teeth, but people's interest and situations evolve. Three consecutive "no" answers might be followed by a "yes" if one's best friend now has sparkling-white teeth, a relationship change has occurred, the individual noticed a few more wrinkles, or recently endured a birthday ending with a damn zero.

If a patient expresses no interest in whiter teeth, the topic is immediately dropped. We make no effort to "sell" whitening, but feel it is our professional duty to make people aware of its availability. (Trust me...many patients don't know little-old-you can perform the marvelous dental techniques they read about in those numerous consumer magazines. The last month I was in practice, I was asked if I did bonding! Only for about the last 20 years. You have to TELL PATIENTS what you can do for them.)

Our total sales pitch, to those who indicate an interest in lighter teeth, is to hold a B-1 Vita shade tab next to their teeth, and let them observe the difference between B-1 and their teeth in a mirror. I explain that we can get their teeth A-1 white, and keep them that way. If they express continued interest--and virtually everyone does--I show them a stint, explain our suggestions for wearing it, and answer their questions.

I've never had a whitening case fail, and this includes one tetracycline case and an 81-year-old female whose teeth were much darker than A-4 when we began. I DO feel I've failed patients when I discover they've wasted money and time on over-the-counter or infomercial products, with poorly fitting trays, that may be risky to their oral health, and usually don't get the job done.

All our staff have lightened their teeth. This is a service provided by the practice at no charge, as I feel it makes them happy, more self-confident, and better ambassadors for fine dentistry. (Doctor, if you don't have white teeth, or aren't interested in getting them, I'd forget about offering this fine service. People with yellowed teeth don't sell much lightening!)

When a lightening case is accepted, our hygiene assistant takes study models, then prepares the whitening stint. Our hygienist inserts the lightening appliance and evaluates the patient every week until we achieve our desired results. **Consult state laws to see what auxiliary functions concerning tooth lightening are legal in your jurisdiction.**

As an incentive for our hygiene assistant--the one who presents the first key whitening question--we pay her a $10 bonus per arch for every whitening case inserted. The assistant makes the stint in the few spare moments she has, so I feel she earns the additional money. A motivated person can easily make an extra $100 per month on whitening cases alone, and be receiving full salary while fabricating them.

Why all this attention devoted to tooth lightening? I believe it is a wonderful service (it's great to see anything that makes patients EXCITED about dental visits) that patients appreciate. It also opens the door for many other cosmetic treatment options. With the marvelous materials available today, almost anyone who so chooses can have a "movie-star smile."

But let's again consider practice compensation, as any viable business must. (I hope thoughts of NET PROFIT are beginning to automatically present themselves with every new topic addressed by now.

THINK BOTTOM LINE, BABY!) The cost of our bleaching kits runs around $45. I have estimated that the time, material and $10 bonus for tray preparation cost our office about $25 per case in other overhead, for a total expense of $45 + $25 = $70. We charge $400 for a bleaching case, making our profit $400 - $70 = $330 per arch treated.

Dentist total time involved is 10 minutes, maximum. (My total commitment involves explaining the process during already scheduled examination times, either for new patients or recare.) Since I can complete 6 cases in one hour, our **average hourly profit per bleaching case** is 6 x $330 = **$1,980**!!!

Any office that has implemented competent systems can average 10 lightening cases per month, for a ($330 x 10 =) $3,300 increase in NET PROFIT. And I've never had a whitening case where the patient wasn't pleased with my results. (I don't know about your practice, but I've had folks less than thrilled about the ultimate outcome of every other type of procedure I perform.)

Our hygiene assistant also exposes the majority of FMX we require for all periodontal patients. (We use a Panorex routinely, but demand an FMX for C, D and F perio patients.) She also takes routine bitewings, Panorex and PAX, as indicated by the dentists. As we'll examine more completely in a moment, our hygiene assistant's ancillary production--those tasks done outside of pure perio--more than pays for her salary. (Expanded hygiene in an efficient office just keeps on giving!)

Expanded Hygiene Assistant Duties

Besides polishing, flossing, administering fluoride treatments, taking x-rays, performing chart audit calls (discussed in a following segment) and the routine tasks we've already discussed, I'd like to mention additional ways in which our hygiene assistant's efforts add value to our office.

We frequently ask her to take orthodontic records (these consisting of a Panorex and cephalometric film, study models with bite, and seven photos). We also ask her to take routine study models for ortho, C & B, and removable cases.

I've always enjoyed the challenge of fabricating dentures and partials. When done efficiently, this care can be very lucrative, and providing such treatment never causes pain! (I find that fact a refreshing change of pace!) Having the luxury of an in-house lab, run by an experienced, skilled and motivated laboratory technician (thanks Larry!) allows me to complete denture cases within a week, and has increased my appreciation of, and skill with, removable prosthodontics.

NOTHING a dentist does can enhance the existence of a patient as much as replacing an unacceptable set of poorly fitting, ugly, ill-biting complete dentures with one that restores health, beauty and function. Such a metamorphosis can truly enhance the quality of a patient's life.

There exists a block of time each morning and afternoon, just as Melissa begins treatment on her first patient, when we have an open chair in hygiene and 20 to 30 minutes of hygiene assistant time available. (The length of time depends on the amount of scale time Melissa has scheduled for her patient.)

Melissa is also willing to occasionally finish treatment on her last patient of the morning or afternoon, freeing up another segment of hygiene assistant time. All production by the hygiene assistant is recorded and paid as hygiene productivity, which makes the unfailingly pleasant Melissa even more willing to let her assistant work independently. (You may have correctly guessed, I'm not one who likes to see anyone I'm paying have nothing to do. Idle hands are the devil's tools...at least according to my grandmother. Personally, the majority of my wicked ideas generally involve entirely different organ systems!)

Having a chairside's assistance during treatment of advanced periodontal disease (and placement of sealants), to ensure an ideally clean field by rinsing, suctioning and retracting tissue, is essential to optimal hygienist efficiency and performance. As you know, heavy bleeding accompanies this level of periodontal treatment. Performing care without an assistant would be akin to the dentist removing an impacted tooth solo. It could be done, but who would want to???

Likewise, periodontal charting can be completed in half the time, with enhanced accuracy, if an assistant enters pocket depths into our computer, as they are called out by the hygienist.

In Iowa, an assistant can perform a toothbrush and prophy-cup fluoride. (Of course, no one but a licensed hygienist or dentist can remove calculus, and any child with even the slightest tartar buildup is scheduled for a prophylaxis with Melissa.) For child fluorides, we disclose kids' teeth, have them brush away all discernible debris under our supervision (thus adding OHI to the service), then polish ONLY any remaining stained areas the brushing failed to remove before administering topical fluoride.

Pumice removes a small portion of the super-hard outer layer of enamel, so we avoid polishing already caries-prone kids' teeth unless visible stain is present. Hygiene assistants and chairsides both perform these preventive fluoride treatments in our office, based on who's available, and what is most convenient.

For example, if a child requires some restorative care, my assistant might perform the fluoride at the end of our treatment, saving the family an additional trip to our office, while enhancing office efficiency and profitability. Setting up and breaking down rooms is expensive and time-consuming. Since OSHA became such a prominent portion of dentistry's vocabulary, we work even harder to require as few patient visits as possible to complete needed care. Busy families also greatly appreciate our efficiency.

Our hygiene assistant also duplicates x-rays for insurance companies, referrals to specialists or for patients leaving our practice. (We never send original films!!) She also makes custom trays for fixed and removable prosthodontic cases, and, as mentioned previously, tooth lightening stints.

Don't let this wonderful array of skills disguise the fact that the hygiene assistant's main reason to exist is **to optimize patient relationships, answer every patient's questions, and be certain each patient feels special attention was given to him or her during recare visits. Hygiene assistant is primarily a people-skill, communication-intensive position. However, if our talented hygiene assistant can create extra income for the practice, and help us in other valuable ways at the same time, so much the better.**

Let's proceed to analyze additional statistics we employ to enhance our hygiene department's performance. I know numbers can be dull and, to some, intimidating. They used to be for me too, until I realized that to strengthen any business, one must vividly understand that **numbers represent the road-map to riches!**

Since the 1986 Tax REFORM (Ha, Ha) Act, it has become almost impossible to achieve wealth through earned income. The great majority of my net worth is the result of investing saved earnings, in as tax-wise a manner as possible, primarily in individual stocks. To be a successful investor, or to run a successful business--like a dental office--one must discern the critical lessons hidden within that entity's numbers.

Chapter 4

Hygiene Monitors and Recruitment

I monitor our office's essential functions with the same intensity with which a conscientious physician would oversee the vital signs of a beloved patient. As I've mentioned, these figures--dry and boring for so many--I consider to be a map to riches. (Lest you forget...I'm pro-riches!)

But I'm not the only member of our team concerned with these indispensable figures. At every month's staff meeting, copies of our five pages of office data are handed to each staff member, and thoroughly reviewed by our team as a group. My staff understands that their individual success depends upon the overall achievement of the practice. (If they didn't, they wouldn't be a team.) Thus they are extremely interested to see how well our monitors indicated we have kept our office ship on course toward our mutual goals.

In addition to specific hygiene monitors, kept by the hygiene team itself (that we'll discuss later in this chapter), approximately one-fourth of the first page of overall office monitors deals with hygiene. I have reproduced the hygiene portion of our total office monitors for 1999 here for your perusal.

HYGIENE MONITORS FOR 1999

	Jan	Feb	Mar	Apr	May	Jun	Jul	Aug	Sep	Oct	Nov	Dec
1 Melissa Production	11,670.76	13,397.81	15,230.24	17,019.49	17,213.74	11,114.81	13,204.96	18,941.26	13,422.00	17,068.56	12,555.67	12,431.50
2 Days wkd / Hr	$12\frac{1}{4}$ / 97	$11\frac{1}{3}$ / 91	14 / 111	$16\frac{1}{2}$ / 132	$16\frac{1}{4}$ / 130	12 / 94	12 / 95	$17\frac{1}{2}$ / 140	13 / 101	$15\frac{3}{4}$ / 134	$12\frac{1}{2}$ / 99	10 / 90
3 Prod/Hr	$120	$147	$137	$129	$132	$118	$139	$135	$133	$127	$126	$138
4 # Patients	152	156	196	219	200	155	165	249	165	214	159	143
5 YTD Production	11,670.76	25,068.57	40,298.81	57,318.30	74,532.04	85,646.85	98,851.81	117,793.07	131,215.00	148,283.00	160,838.67	173,270.17
6 Days wkd / Hr	$12\frac{1}{4}$ / 97	$23\frac{1}{2}$ / 188	$37\frac{1}{2}$ / 299	54 / 431	$70\frac{1}{4}$ / 561	$82\frac{1}{4}$ / 655	$94\frac{1}{4}$ / 750	$111\frac{3}{4}$ / 890	$124\frac{3}{4}$ / 991	$140\frac{1}{2}$ / 1117	153 / 1216	163 / 1306
7 Prod / Hr	$120	$133	$135	$133	$133	$131	$132	$132	$134	$132	$132	$133
8 # Patients	152	308	504	723	923	1078	1243	1492	1593	1807	1966	2109
	Jan	Feb	Mar	Apr	May	Jun	Jul	Aug	Sep	Oct	Nov	Dec

Consider January, 1999.

Line 1 records Melissa's production for the month, totaling $11,670.76.

Line 2 reveals the number of days worked (12 1/4) and hours of patient care provided (97).

Line 3 shows the statistic I find most critical--average production per hour, here listed as $120. (Derived by dividing production $11,670.76 by hours worked 97.)

Days and hours worked vary greatly from month to month. In 1999, a low of 90 hours was worked in December, a high of 140 hours in August. This extreme divergence makes total production figures per month almost meaningless. However, **average hourly production accurately reflects efficiency of care delivery**, no matter how slightly or prodigiously we labored, and this is what most concerns me.

Line 4 reveals the number of patients seen that month to be 152.

Lines 5 through 8 are running totals or averages for the year-to-date. In January, they are identical for the month and year-to-date. (DAH!)

Please skip to the far right, under December, and let's consider some data there. Line 1 shows production for that month was $12,431.50, this treatment occurring (line 2) during 10 days or 90 hours of offered care. Average hourly production for the month was $138, with 143 (low for the year) patients seen.

Beginning on December's line 5, we see total hygiene production for 1999 was $173,270.17. This was accomplished in 163 days, or 1306 hours. Average hourly production for the year was $133.

We've discussed these results previously, but I felt being able to review the source of the data--our monitors--might prove helpful to those motivated souls willing to track their own journey, and possibly be of some interest to the rest.

The entire five pages of general office monitors are reviewed in painstaking detail (it was painful to write it all--refer to line 11, under August. Ugh!) in Chapter 4 of *Dentistry's Future*. The portion of our hygiene monitors reproduced here represents less than 5 percent of the total office information regularly compiled and reviewed. This lengthy chapter in *Future* is probably not too thrilling to read either, but the enlightened understand that tremendous productivity rewards those who chart precise paths, then monitor their progress, and make adjustments as feedback indicates.

Hygiene Monitors

1	Date	Canc	Filled	Fail	Filled	Open	Filled	Total
2	2	0	0	0	0	0	0	0
3	3	0	0	40	0	0	0	40
4	4	40	40	30	30	30	30	0
5	5	30	0	0	0	0	0	30
6	6	0	0	0	0	0	0	0
7	9	30	30	90	60	0	0	30
8	10	0	0	0	0	0	0	0
9	11	0	0	40	0	0	0	40
10	13	30	0	0	0	0	0	30
11	16	40	40	50	30	30	40	10
12	17	20	20	0	0	0	0	0
13	18	0	0	0	0	0	0	0
14	19	30	0	90	0	0	0	120
15	23	30	30	50	0	0	0	50
16	24	0	0	70	0	0	0	70
17	25	0	0	70	0	0	0	70
18	26	70	0	0	0	0	0	70
19	28	0	0	70	0	0	0	70
20	18 days	160		480		over 10 minutes		630
21		8.9 min		26.7 min				630/18 days =
		canc per day		failed per day				35 min
								35 min lost per day

FEBRUARY HYGIENE MONITORS

In addition to the five 17 by 11-inch pages of general office monitors, our hygiene assistant generates internal monitors for hygiene staff and my edification. These are reviewed during the hygiene staff meeting, which immediately follows the entire office staff meeting each month. Individuals involved in the gathering include myself, Melissa, her assistant and the member of the front office team whose primary duty it is to handle hygiene scheduling. (One front office person, of the three who work there, is always assigned hygiene scheduling as her PRINCIPAL task.)

Please consider our February monitor for unfilled hygiene time. Begin by examining Line 3, which illustrates that on February 3, there was 0 cancelled (canc) hygiene minutes (of which 0 were filled). There was 40 minutes of failed (fail) time, all of which remained unfilled, and 0 minutes of open (or unscheduled) time (of which 0 was filled). Thus for the entire day (under total), 40 minutes of hygiene time was unproductive.

Line 4, February 4, illustrates 40 minutes of canceled time was filled, 30 minutes of failed time was filled and 30 unscheduled minutes were also filled, so from the entire 100 minutes of possible wasted time that occurred that day, no open time (0 under total) remained in our hygiene department.

You can bet the front office staff mentioned this significant feat to Melissa and me, probably several times! You'd also be safe in wagering that Melissa and I were delighted that 100 minutes of her valuable time became productive due to the diligent and adroit efforts of our excellent team!

This is a propitious moment to reflect on the likely scenario within your office if 100 minutes of hygiene time became unscheduled, for a variety of reasons, during the course of any given day. How much of this limited resource (hygiene time) would you estimate was likely to be filled, and **if you don't keep monitors, how would you know?**

Before hygiene was paid based on production, I'd guess a couple of calls would have been made, but I can almost guarantee little of this 100 minutes of open time would have been scheduled in my office, posing a severe threat of potential hygienist caffeine overdose. Now that our hygienist's salary is on the line, someone besides myself has a vested interest in maximizing hygiene production. I like that a lot!

Skip to Line 7, February 9, where 90 minutes of failure occurred, 60 of which was filled, leaving 30 minutes (total) of the day open. See how this works?

Line 21 is the month's summary. An average of 8.9 minutes of cancelled time, 26.7 minutes of failed time and virtually zero minutes of unfilled time (unfilled for the month was actually over-booked by 10 minutes, probably a 30-scale patient placed in a 20-scale opening, which happens) existed each day of this month, for a composite 35 minutes of open time per hygiene day worked in February.

Often a 40-minute scaling appointment will be filled on short notice by a patient requiring only 30 minutes of hygienist time, so 10 minutes will remain unfilled, and accurately recorded as unscheduled time--a problem with which Melissa and I can survive. Even I don't begrudge an occasional 10-minute break!

MEASURED BEHAVIOR IMPROVES. We keep monitors concerning appointment slots successfully filled to assess our team's aptitude at the difficult task of filling open time on a hygiene schedule which occurs that day. (It's more enjoyable to monitor and discuss time filled, rather than discussing only unfilled and thus wasted time!)

To help fill short-notice open time, we offer a 10 percent discount on all hygiene fees for someone willing to be treated on the day we have open time available. We have nurtured a small community of stay-home folks--basically comprised of the retired population and moms with all children in school--who expect to be called on short notice, and appreciate this price break. We, in turn, are delighted to fill this open time with 90 percent of normal production, as even with my rudimentary math skills, I understand 90 percent is more than zero!

This "short notice" list is kept in a "tickler file," separated by month of patient's next suggested recare. **We don't appoint these patients in advance**, as we've previously gained their permission to be scheduled in such a manner. They expect and appreciate our discounted short-notice appointments. (Some folks just love a bargain, and a goodly number of those people are retired, or raising young families. I also think they enjoy our gratitude and expressions of thanks-always forthcoming--for helping us with the difficult and time-consuming task of filling short-notice cancellations.)

Of course, we are professionally obligated to be certain none of these patients slip beyond their ideal recall intervals. But with 48 (12 per day x 4 days) or so hygiene opportunities available per week, I doubt we've ever had a single week that didn't require us to fill numerous openings. Our valuable "short-notice" club makes this sometimes challenging task much easier and more pleasant. (Doctor, ask your front desk people if they have EVER had a patient THRILLED to fill a short-term cancellation, as our 10-percent-off folks are. Success is all about consistently doing things in the most efficient possible manner, i.e., creating excellent systems.)

As helpful as this strategy has been, whenever possible Melissa and I would prefer to limit the discounted care we offer, and fill time in other, 100% productive ways. To help fill openings for which we have over 24-hour notice, unfilled hygiene times for the next several days are posted on a piece of paper hung next to the master schedule posted in our hallway. (An example of such a note might be "40 scale open at 3 P.M. Friday.") Thus the entire staff is aware of time available, and can help fill these openings from among the patients they treat.

Often an additional visit to our practice is saved by our awareness, as a patient already in the office for other care needs a prophy and we can provide it that day. The patient is as grateful for our consideration as we are for the additional opportunity to provide care.

Emergency patients, usually overdue for preventive care, and frequently motivated by their recent problems, are another possible source of appointments for care within the next few days.

Now let's review the hygiene annual summary monitors.

DECEMBER YEAR-TO-DATE HYGIENE MONITORS

	Days Worked	Cancel	Fail	Open	Total Loss
January	19	23.3	23.6	0	46.9 min
February	18	7.2	28.8	0	36.0 min
March	18	12.7	38.8	0	51.5 min
April	22	9.5	16.4	6.4	32.3 min
May	23	17.4	23	7.8	48.2 min
June	17	5.3	18.2	1.8	25.3 min
July	17	8.8	35.9	9.4	54.1 min
August	21	5.7	22.9	21.0	49.6 min
September	21	13.3	21	35.7	70.0 min
October	22	11.4	5.9	18.6	35.9 min
November	18	4.4	22.8	3.3	30.5 min
December	17	6.5	20.6	0	27.1 min
Yr to Date Total	233 days	125.5	277.9	104.0	507.4 min
Average Month	19.4	6.5 min cancel	14.3 min fail	5.3 min open	26.1 min lost

Our year-to-date hygiene monitor shows an average of 6.5 minutes of cancelled time, 14.3 minutes of failed appointments and 5.3 minutes of open or unscheduled time, for a total annual average of 26.1 minutes of open time per day. When one begins to monitor, an average below 40 open minutes a day is excellent. One might review his or her office's preceding past few months of hygiene records and calculate how much open time existed, on an average daily basis, in one's own situation, to establish a baseline for comparison. This data shouldn't prove too hard for a staff member to retrieve from old day sheets.

I predict most dentists paying their hygienist a fixed salary--whether hourly, weekly or monthly--are going to receive an unpleasant surprise when faced with accurate totals of non-productive time. I suspect most dentists don't keep track of unproductive hygiene time, because, due to the amount of salary paid to hygienists, they just don't want to know how much time and money was wasted. It's often painful to view the unvarnished truth, but there is power in knowledge, when the acquired wisdom is ACTED UPON.

Hygiene production is basically determined by the fullness of the schedule. Although D and F periodontal treatment, sealants and tooth lightening are more lucrative, the large, high-revenue cases possible for dentists don't exist in hygiene. This is why, to be optimally productive, one must carefully control unfilled hygiene time, and why we monitor this finite and precious commodity (time) to one-tenth of a minute! Let's consider how we handle unscheduled time, based on the particular reason it exists.

We require 24-hour notice for changes in appointments. It says so right on the appointment card! If **cancelled day of** openings were a problem, it might indicate we'd grown negligent about reminding patients of our long-standing two failures or two same-day cancellations policy, after which such unfortunate events, **patients will be dismissed from the practice!**

Every patient is advised of this failure policy (I love baseball-I'm a huge White Sox fan--but in our office the rule is two strikes and you're out), in a gentle way, before their first examination appointment. (Explaining this BEFORE a failure occurs is nothing personal, merely an explanation of existing policy. Having to discuss the matter AFTER a failure can come across as threatening and punitive.) We make exceptions to this rule for long-standing patients with reliable histories, or for those whom the staff believes have creditable excuses, but good patients failing, and true emergencies forcing cancellations, are rare events.

I don't want to be paid a fee for a failed appointment. I want the chronic-failure people out of my life! I'm sure God loves them, but my life is too short to deal with undependable or disingenuous people. In reality, those who don't show up are NOT patients. They're just names on a schedule that become non-production profit-stripping holes in our day.

If **failed** time was increasing, we might concentrate on confirming all appointments **directly with the patient**, being sure not to just leave messages on machines or with other people. It's okay to leave a notice, so long as the message is "please call our office to confirm your reserved time."

We confirm all appointments at least 24 hours in advance. Every confirmed patient has a small (c) placed by their name on our master day-sheet. Any patient scheduled that day and not marked confirmed is called by our hygiene assistant immediately after our morning clearing and huddle, while the hygienist begins her first patient's care. (If the assistant is busy with a patient immediately, she asks the front-office team to make any needed calls during the course of our morning huddle.)

We would also reaffirm that we are continuing to do an excellent job of stressing the critical importance of timely recare while patients are in the office. However, when hygienists are paid on commission, I don't believe you'll find failure to emphasize the significance of periodontal maintenance to be a problem. Again, hygienists aren't paid if patients don't return. Such bare-bones reality has always motivated me.

If **unscheduled** time was a concern, chart audit or new patient recruitment might require one's attention. Methods to enhance patient volume will be covered in a following segment.

Hygiene also keeps one additional sheet of monitors for their own information. (Remember, numbers are maps to riches!)

HYGIENE MONITOR THREE

		White & Bright	Rota-dent	Pt has Rota-dent
February	2	1	1	1
	3	1	2	1
	4	1	1	0
	5	1	2	1
	6	1	3	1
	9	2	2	1
	10	2	3	0
	11	1	2	0
	13	1	1	0
	16	2	3	1
	17	0	3	2
	18	0	3	0
	19	0	3	0
	23	0	2	0
	24	0	2	0
	26	2	2	2
	28	0	1	0
	Total	15	36	10

Studying the February chart, one can see 15 White and Bright treatments were suggested and discussed, 36 Rota-dents recommended and 10 patients seen who were already using a Rota-dent. The topics evaluated by this monitor are determined by Melissa and her assistant, and are based on the premise that **measured behavior improves**. (I trust this important truism is beginning to have a familiar ring.) The hygiene department monitors whatever facet of hygiene treatment they most wish to see enhanced, and their targets vary as time passes.

For several months they monitored how many warm face towels were handed out, to develop the habit of using this value-added service when the machine was new to our office. (I purchased a special machine to warm towels. Today I'd use a Crock Pot to get the job done, as preparing towels this way is simple, cheap and easy. Most patients do enjoy a warm, moist, lemon-scented towel to refresh themselves with after receiving care.)

Monitoring how many patients had images displayed on hygiene's intra-oral camera, or number of tooth lightening cases suggested versus accepted, might be worth considering.

Hygiene Recruitment

There exists no advantage to believing in, and being committed to, an outstanding, profitable hygiene department, if a dentist can't discover and employ an excellent hygienist to share one's dream and accomplishments. I believe every dentist can identify and hire this key staff person, if he or she is properly motivated by understanding the philosophy we've been discussing, and accepting how critical hygiene is to overall patient oral health and practice financial success. If a doctor is thus aware, he or she will pursue a hygienist with a zeal similar in intensity to that with which the drowning seek air!

As a personal credo, I don't accept "can't" from myself or those around me. I do allow "It isn't worth my trouble," or, "I'm too lazy," as these statements are true. My kids are sick of my rejection of their explanations of why something wasn't done with a dismissive wave of my hand and the affirmation that "People do what they truly desire to do." Any excuses offered beyond this truism are merely defensive B.S. and pathetic attempts at self-delusion.

People committed to maximizing their health exercise. Those dedicated to optimal oral health floss. The uncommitted find a plethora of justifications--none of them their fault--to excuse their failure to perform acts they know to be in their best interests. "People do what they truly desire to do."

I've never been without a hygienist for more than a few weeks, and that single opening was many years ago, and probably was the critical event that led to the creation of my high-powered hygiene recruiting system. As you'll soon witness, I leave no opportunity unexamined in my hygienist quest. I understand--as by now does every reader--how essential productive hygiene is to my office.

Let's first consider doing what everyone else does when they need a hygienist--only performing it better--before examining a few more original efforts. What follows is the ad we place in dental journals or area newspapers:

Dental Hygienist

Are you kind, compassionate, people-oriented and motivated to succeed? We are seeking an exceptional person for our progressive office. We focus on warmth, caring and expert communication with our patients. We emphasize personal development through continuing education, full participation with other team members and high involvement with clients. Applicants should be career-minded, personally stable and health-centered in their lifestyles. If you are searching for a real opportunity to grow and fulfill your potential, please call us at 319-524-8811.

John A. Wilde, D.D.S., P.C., and Staff
1610 Morgan Street
Keokuk, Iowa 52632.

Every aspect of staff recruitment is covered in great detail in Chapter 9 of *Bringing Your Practice Into Focus*. All the forms, including applications, phone interviews, patterned personal interviews, and critical **reference checks** we employ when filling any staff opening are reproduced there in full. To make this book a stand-alone resource, I've placed our standard hiring forms, along with my comments regarding their optimal use, in the appendix. Our hiring system--which allows us to identify the best possible job candidate--is a critical portion of our practice success.

Since I usually have only one hygienist applicant, our customary evaluation system for potential team members isn't as important for hygienists (and this is why I delegated this otherwise crucial information to the appendix), but the protocol is invaluable for other staff hirings, including hygiene assistant.

Despite our process's limited application in hygiene hiring (due to usually having only one applicant), please understand that nothing is more critical to practice success than staff, and I take great pains to optimize EVERY hiring, including the person who daily cleans our office.

Dixie, our cleaning lady for a decade, is an equal partner in our bonus system, and is involved in all office social functions. She's a neat lady, whose work-hardened and time-tested values I admire, and a spotless office is an integral factor in positive patient perception. (If there's dust on your reception area lamp, patients will question how well you sterilize equipment, and who can blame them for such concerns?)

The first vital step in any hiring is identifying qualified people and motivating them to contact one's office. (With approximately 30 Iowa-schooled graduates a year shared among 1,400 Iowa dentists, this is especially true for hygienists.)

Notice our ad avoids all the usual topics and assertions--good pay, benefits, hours, boss doesn't have too much B.O.--and **focuses entirely on value and character**. I don't desire to hire just a body with a hygiene certificate! I want the special person described in the advertisement to be the one offering periodontal therapy in my exceptional office. I hope this ad will intrigue hygienists who aren't actively seeking a job, but may not be completely happy or satisfied in their current office. (Reading *RDH* leaves one with the inescapable conclusion that the numbers of dissatisfied hygienists are legion!)

This ad is placed in all the customary places like *RDH*, 918-831-9742, *JADA*, 800-621-8099, and every nearby state dental journal.

It often takes two to three months for these advertisements to be published, and I rarely have the luxury of such time to replace a departing hygienist. However, I'd rather waste a few hundred dollars on these advertisements, and have a hygienist already in place when the ads run, than risk still not having a hygienist two months after an opening occurs, and belatedly placing the ads then.

The profit potential of our hygiene department makes running the ads an easy decision. There's always the possibility, even if one is fortunate enough to have found a hygienist before these notices first see light of day, that the new hygienist-office relationship has not proven to be ideal, and additional applicants would be welcome.

I've also placed these notices in the want-ad section of every major city paper within 250 miles of our office (including Chicago, St. Louis, Kansas City and Des Moines). This is expensive! In the two times I've run these advertisements in metropolitan newspapers, I've yet to receive a single response; however, I'd try this approach again, if I was desperate. (I generally need only one applicant to make my efforts a success.)

Our hygienist before Melissa gave us one week's notice. This makes dentist and staff a little tense (more precisely, RIGID!), when patients are booked solid for the entire year! (How would you enjoy calling and cancelling thousands of appointments?) Melissa was working part-time for us then and, to our delight, left her other office and was working full-time in our practice within two weeks. She made this decision, despite the fact that she lives **90 miles from our practice**. Her dedication is such that she completed this arduous journey for over four years, rarely ever missing a day, or even being a few minutes late.

If one lived in or near an urban area (where one hunts what? pigeons?), a city newspaper want ad might prove successful. Local dental or hygiene societies might also be of significant assistance in metropolitan settings. Unfortunately, these ain't much help out here in the sticks.

Some New Twists on Ways to Locate a Hygienist

So much for what everyone else does. Now let's deal with the more unique methods I employ whereby almost every hygienist I've ever hired has been recruited. (The following techniques require some staff time to implement, but are ultimately much quicker to achieve results, and are relatively inexpensive!)

Most state hygienist associations will provide anyone who requests it with a list--complete with addresses and phone numbers-of every member of their organization. In my experience, it's a bit hard to track these groups down. No established business office exists. Usually, one has to reach the society's president at home after work. But the lists are inexpensive, as I assume the associations are motivated to offer them in an effort to help identify employment opportunities for their members.

The ADA (phone number 800-621-8099) also provides an inexpensive book listing every hygiene school in America, along with the name of the hygiene department head, plus address, phone, fax and e-mail information. (The American Association of Dental Schools--202-667-9433--is also a rich source of information concerning dental education facilities.)

We send the following letter to every hygienist listed by state societies, and to every student in each hygiene school within our 250-mile radius of interest:

Dear ,

We are in need of a Dental Hygienist to join our strongly team-oriented dental practice. Our staff is dedicated to helping each other grow as individuals, and fulfilling not just the dental needs, but the human needs of our patients. We are seeking a people-oriented individual who desires to develop personally and professionally.

Ours is a general dentistry practice in which care from all dental specialties is included. We are strongly preventive and periodontally oriented, treating advanced periodontal cases. We encourage use of sealants, recommend fluoride aggressively and stress each patient's achieving and maintaining optimum oral health.

Our office is fully computerized (nine (9) terminals), and features five (5) fully equipped operatories, all with their own x-rays, Nitrous Oxide, intra-oral cameras and virtual reality glasses. Two of these completely equipped rooms are reserved for the use of our hygienist and her assistant exclusively.

Our staff of three (3) dentists, three (3) chairsides (including expanded-hygiene assistant) and three (3) front-office staff are committed to providing the highest quality of care for our over 5,000 patients of record.

We are located in Keokuk, Iowa, a town of 13,000, located on the banks of the Mississippi on the extreme southeast tip of Iowa. We are 95 miles south of Iowa City, and midway between Burlington, Iowa, and Quincy, Illinois.

Keokuk is a typically friendly Iowa community, with an excellent YMCA and downtown mall. The area is sports- and family-oriented, with a mixture of businesses (there exists no one large employer whose labor problems could threaten office prosperity), and a relaxed, rural flavor.

We appreciate your assistance in our quest for a qualified and motivated individual. This is an outstanding opportunity for the right person, and we look forward to hearing from you soon.

Sincerely,

John A. Wilde, D.D.S., P.C., and Staff

(Please feel free to copy or adapt any information in this book for your personal use. Imitation is the most sincere form of flattery!)

As stated, this letter is mailed to every member of the state hygiene association, and to every hygiene school. I personally contact the head of each hygiene school in our tri-state area of Iowa, Illinois and Missouri about a week after the letters are mailed. (I believe speaking directly to a person in authority creates a much stronger impression than merely sending a letter, or asking a factotum to call.) Often the school's dean is aware of a graduate looking for work, or has an idea of a possible suitable candidate, perhaps among past graduates.

The dean will usually agree to place a copy of our letter in each student's mailbox. We also send photos of our office to each hygiene school, featuring our two fully equipped and beautiful hygiene rooms, to place in their job-opening files, along with a reproduction of the above letter.

After two weeks, if we've not had several calls expressing interest, either I personally, or (almost always) a key, experienced member of my staff will contact by phone each member of the state hygiene association to whom we've sent a letter, greet them warmly, inquire if they have any interest in our opportunity and answer their questions. Sometimes the person we call isn't interested, but can direct us to another hygienist who he or she has heard might be considering changing jobs. (Not all hygienists are constituents of their societies, and I know of no organized method to contact nonmembers.)

It is imperative that a key staff member coordinate all these recruiting efforts, and be allowed enough time away from her customary duties to perform this important task to the utmost of her abilities. Most of the hygienists we contact are currently working, so they must be reached after five P.M. Special arrangements must be made concerning working hours of the team member making these important calls. (She might need permission to take mornings off, or receive authorization for overtime.) I don't care how long this calling takes, and I don't want the job rushed!! A team member taking the time to build a relationship with a possible hygienist might be the key to his or her accepting an interview. Once they tour our facility, peruse our fiscal results, and meet our team, I have every confidence we can hire them.

Except for the first time I developed this system, the only step in hygiene recruiting in which I'm personally involved is calling the deans of the various hygiene schools. This job takes about 90 minutes. Of course, I conduct interviews personally.

I've never failed to identify a qualified applicant by the combination of these methods. Yes, it's a lot of work and somewhat expensive. If that concerns you, you may be suffering a short-term memory problem! Please flip back to review the figures detailing our net profit from hygiene.

As I stated, application forms, patterned interview, etc. are provided in this book's appendix. I would caution every dentist to **always perform reference checks on any staff member one is considering employing, including associate dentists and hygienists.** I've heard many horror stories concerning staff embezzlement, alcohol, drug, and other personal problems of a severe nature--all clearly identified in the previous place of employment--if only the new employer had taken a few moments to investigate.

Our staff is carefully coached to provide no information beyond dates of employment, and beginning and ending salary, concerning inquiries about any of our previous team members. To volunteer more puts one at legal risk!!! Fortunately, most dental offices aren't aware of this, and especially if one calls staff at home, he or she-including dentists--will often be extremely candid in their comments. Little information is more valuable to the hiring process than knowing how past co-workers viewed your prospective employee. The key question is, "Would you hire him or her again?"

I've twice been approached by area dentists seeking to relocate, and asked to consider purchasing their practices. (Although I've been tempted, I've never done so. I like to say opening a satellite office was the one mistake in dentistry I never got around to making.)

When carefully evaluating a dental business opportunity, I consider high hygiene profit to be more important than dentist's production. This notable assertion seems to have escaped the awareness of most. Allow me to explain my reasoning.

Time is the most precious commodity of anyone involved in any service industry. (We are all rather limited by that 24 hours in a day thing.) Any source of added revenue that doesn't require the practice owner's active involvement--that in effect allows him or her to leverage available time--is immensely important.

That critical reality is why so much of *Dentistry's Future* is devoted to the possibilities of enhanced income, with less time in office, by employing associates. (Recall my data from 1996, when I saw patients for 52 eight-hour days, and averaged a daily net of $6,673. This highly profitable result is how the ability to leverage one's time appears on a Profit and Loss statement.) The capability to magnify dentists' profits, without investing more of their time, is what makes expanded hygiene so important to ultimate fiscal results.

I'm an active investor, and am always considering ways to further enhance my flow of unearned income. But, no matter how promising an opportunity might appear, I avoid any business venture that involves much of my time after it's initially established. If one must commit his or her time to make money on a project, it's a job, not an investment. Most dentists have jobs aplenty!

My professional goal was to create an office of highly refined, effective and efficient **systems**, that could run extremely well **when I wasn't there**. Excellent expanded hygiene is one such critical revenue source that is available to any dentist, even those who choose not to face the more daunting hassles inherent in associate relationships.

This brief segment will give you a chance to meet--at least on the written page--our wonderful hygienist, Melissa Lannery R.D.H. Her office nickname was Sunshine, and better than anyone I've ever met, she pulled off an almost impossible trifecta. Melissa was great with people, highly skilled technically and extremely timely and organized. Few in any profession excel in all major facets of their chosen work. I've stated many times that I could only wish to live up to my hygienist's level of professionalism.

Her final assistant, Linda, was not with our office that long, but she was delightful, energetic and always brightened our day. I miss them both.

I asked Melissa to write a brief note explaining her unique take on expanded hygiene, as I felt hygienists could better relate to her words. We have examined enough benefits for you to realize that she could have written about efficiency or production. Typical of Melissa, she chose to discuss how working as a team benefits all involved.

Melissa pokes a little fun at me. That illustrates the typical flavor of our office. You can joke with people you trust and like. But, it can't be just the dentist teasing, or it comes across--as it most likely is--as bullying.

A Note from Melissa

I had the wonderful opportunity of working in John's office with the expanded hygiene program for about five years. Now, before joining John's office, I had never worked with an assistant, and I wasn't sure exactly what expanded hygiene entailed. And to be truthful, when John explained the program to me, I still kind of thought, "What do I need an assistant for? I'm doing fine just the way things are." But I thought, "Let's give it a try." And it wasn't long after getting into it that I had to admit John actually knew what he was talking about. (An admission I would reluctantly have to make many times over our years together.)

I found that I really enjoyed the teamwork approach of my hygiene assistant (named Linda), myself, along with John contributing to patient care. I felt the patient received more personalized care and aspects of care could be emphasized more. For instance, I could let patients know about areas they were missing in their oral hygiene. When Linda came in to do their polishing and flossing she would again point out bleeding areas, what this signified and how to control the problem. When John came in for the examination, he would again reinforce these areas that needed work. This way the patient got three different perspectives and three different ways of approaching the subject and motivating, not just one hygienist giving the typical "lecture." After three different caregivers see and point out the same thing, it begins to soak in.

Another example was as I was working with the patient oftentimes I would point out areas that John had recommended for treatment in the past, or maybe note a new area of concern. I could discuss why treatment was recommended with the patient. When Linda came in she would take an intra-oral picture of the area, discuss it with the patient and the groundwork was laid for John to diagnose treatment.

Again patients had three different people taking an active role in their care, and three different perspectives on how and why something needed to be done. This was often very helpful, as everyone has a different personality, and different approaches work for different interests. My way of explaining may get through to one patient, but maybe Linda's personality was more suited to get through to the next patient. (Editor's note: John also has a personality...if not an especially pleasant one!) So where one left off, another picked up.

Therefore personality was a consideration when looking for a hygiene assistant. Because we would all be working together, we had to find someone whose goal was to work as part of a team. Good time-management skills were important also. The pace was quick and there were many things to do in a set amount of time.

Yet we never wanted the patients to feel as if they were being rushed through. While the patient was there, that was his or her time and no one else's. However, we always strived to stay on schedule. Granted, there were times when special concerns came up which required extra time. And we took it--but we always tried to stay on schedule because we realized that patients' time was just as important as ours.

When circumstances arose that required more time for a patient, it was really beneficial that there were two of us. For instance, if a prophy was taking longer than planned for me, and the next patient was here, Linda would seat them, update the medical history, and take any necessary films--as she usually had already done before I came into the room--then she might take any intra-oral pictures that were going to be needed, discuss areas of concern with the patient and get them pre-booked for their next recall appointment. Or she might just sit and chat with the patient until I got into the room, so the patient wasn't left alone. And for people on the apprehensive side, sitting and chatting with Linda often helped put them at ease. We had also begun to experiment with pre-polishing before my prophy if the patient and Linda were ready before I was. This removed stain and helped me see, and saved us time.

At times Linda needed extra time with the previous patient when I was ready for her. In these instances, I would go ahead and polish, floss, assist during the exam and pre-book the next appointment...whatever needed to be done until she was free. We often helped each other like that, as we worked like partners.

Another quality we looked for in a hygiene assistant was what type of personality she had. We found it advantageous to have a personality that complements our own. Complements, but is not the same as. Where I had downfalls, Linda was strong, and vice versa. There were patient types I could get through to better, and others that related to Linda's approach.

But you definitely needed a people person who is caring and compassionate in patient care. You need someone who's not afraid to tackle subjects with the patients and get in there and show them how it should be done, but in a gentle, caring way.

Working in this type of setting was a real adventure for me. One in which I learned a lot. Unfortunately, John decided to retire, the wimp, so I am no longer in an expanded hygiene setting. After working closely with my assistant for so long it was really difficult to go back to a setting of just the hygienist. I miss the teamwork approach to patient care and all of the advantages it brought with it. Secondly, I miss the partnership between my assistant and myself. (Editor's note: Melissa was probably too emotional to mention how much she MISSED JOHN!)

Sincerely,

Melissa Lannery, R.D.H.

Chapter 5

Soft Tissue Diagnosis and Management: Meeting Today's Standard of Care, While Expanding and Improving Services

by Dr. Herb Bader, D.D.S., F.A.C.D., F.I.C.D.
and Jane Jones, R.D.H.

Pay special attention to the ADDENDUM by Jane at the end of this chapter for a clear, concise ACTION PLAN for PROFITABLE DENTAL HYGIENE.

I felt even my readers deserved a chapter of articulate, intelligent writing, accomplished by acknowledged experts in the field. (I hope you can stand the shock!)

I am deeply indebted to Jane Jones, R.D.H., a delightful and helpful lady, and to Herb Bader, D.D.S., F.A.C.D., F.I.C.D. and all-around nice guy, for the following sweeping, cutting-edge overview of the newest, hottest topics involving periodontal therapy.

Jane Jones has helped hundreds of offices implement and refine Soft Tissue Management during her 37+ year hygiene career. She is a noted educator and lecturer who still practices clinically part time, teaches dental hygiene and develops continuing education programs.

In addition to the Soft Tissue Management courses she gives--teamed with Dr. Bader and a general dentist, Dr. Steve Biagini--throughout the United States and Canada for Pro-Dentec (the company that makes the Rota-dent brush so central to our hygiene success), Ms. Jones presents courses on Chemotherapeutics, Periodontal Debridement, and Recare Systems, Ultrasonics, the New Generation, Maintenance of Periodontal Patients, Implant Maintenance, Hands-on Advanced Scaling and Root Planing with Today's Ultrasonics, and Team Building Through Communication.

Dr. Herb Bader is on staff of the Harvard School of Dental Medicine where he teaches postgraduate periodontics. He completed his postdoctoral training in research, teaching and clinical periodontology at Harvard School of Dental Medicine. (I, on the other hand, have visited Boston once. Bad downtown roads and traffic. I got lost and can't say for certain that I ever did get out.)

Dr. Bader has published a number of articles and abstracts in the field of periodontal diagnosis, and is actively involved in clinical research in that area. He is a **full-time practicing periodontist** in Concord, MA. What follows are Jane Jones, and Dr. Bader's most cogent thoughts. Enjoy!

Periodontal management in the general practice is rapidly moving into a new era of importance and predictability, based on the rapid outpouring of new concepts of the disease mechanism, treatment and long-term management strategies. We are beginning to integrate risk assessment for treatment planning with strong involvement by the hygienist (as part of the team approach), to effectively control the inflammatory phase of periodontitis, prior to decisions regarding the need for further treatment.

To more completely understand our patients, and to more accurately assess their risk for dental disease, a complete medical, medication and supplemental history is taken, along with blood pressure readings and full-mouth series of radiographs with vertical bitewings. Hard and soft tissue exam will include an oral cancer screening, as well as periodontal examination.

The components of a periodontal examination are: tissue observations, presence and location of plaque, calculus and stain, probing depth, bleeding on probing, recession, furcation involvement, fremitus, and mobility.

It is always more effective, as well as efficient, if the hygienist verbally calls out observations to an assistant (or hygiene coordinator or co-therapist) who is recording the data. The patient is more involved in co-examination when the observations are described to the patient before probing, such as what the pocket readings mean, what bleeding means, etc. Patients become a part of the co-discovery, co-examination or co-diagnosis process. The use of intra-oral cameras, or simply a hand mirror, enhances the patient's understanding of the oral condition. A mirror that is mounted on the dental light is also an excellent patient education tool. Some caveats of the examination process are:

1. Always show patients a healthy site first so they can differentiate health from disease in their mouth.
2. Explain the examination prior to the process, and what the "numbers" mean.
3. Explain that bleeding is common but not normal. Healthy gums do not bleed!
4. Recession must be charted, not only because it shows previous

disease, but because it is a more accurate representation of the patient's periodontal status. Many insurance companies do not pay benefits for root planing unless there is at least 4 mm of attachment loss (not just probing depth). Of course, attachment loss is the addition of the pocket measurement plus recession.

There are many different kinds of probes and markings available. Consistency is the most important aspect of the probing technique. Twenty grams of probing pressure is what is taught in hygiene and dental schools as the standard.

Constant pressure probes: There is only one manual probe available that is designed to reference when 20 grams of pressure is used. The Sensor Probe (by Pro-Dentec) has two sections. When they contact, the clinician has applied twenty grams of pressure. This uniformity allows for consistency between operators on the same patient. The clinician actually establishes a rhythm while probing, making the use of this probe very comfortable for both patient and operator. These probes are very cost-effective, available with different markings, and may be autoclaved multiple times.

Electronic probes: The introduction of electronic probes in the mid-1980's stimulated the interest in probing all our patients, while providing excellent graphics of the periodontal chart. The Florida Probe (Florida Probe Corporation, Gainesville, Florida) is probably the most familiar. There are two models, with the initial unit being larger, and featuring computer interface. The smaller new TS-2000 model has a touch-screen capability. Both have data entry through a foot control pedal, or keyboard, with additional features available a la carte, depending upon the individual office's needs. The probe is calibrated to 0.2 mm, which is why this instrument is frequently used in research. The program automatically stores data onto a disk that may be printed out for the patient.

Probe One (The Dental Probe, Inc., Richmond, Virginia) is another similar electronic probe available, and can also interface with a computer. This is an important feature of these types of probes in today's computerized dental offices, and they have the ability to integrate into existing systems. This probe also has a foot control, and is available in different systems to enhance compatibility with existing hardware and software in the office. While the Florida Probe has titanium probe tips, the Probe One has disposable plastic tips. Although both electronic probes promote one-operator convenience, ease of use, and patient comfort, the cost, which is appreciable, will determine their practical application in any given dental office.

These risk assessment and management strategies begin with dentists understanding the current accepted model for periodontal disease is based upon the interaction of the host immune mechanism and putative pathogens. The 1999 World Workshop on Current Classification of Periodontal Disease[1] effected many changes in nomenclature:

I. Gingival Disease (with Sub-classifications)
II. Chronic Periodontitis (Localized or Generalized)
III. Aggressive Periodontitis (Localized or Generalized)
IV. Periodontitis as Manifestation of Systemic Disease
V. Necrotizing Periodontal Disease
VI. Abscesses of the Periodontium
VII. Periodontitis Associated with Endodontic Lesions
VIII. Developmental or Acquired Deformities and Conditions

As is shown here, both gingivitis and periodontitis are divided

[1] *Annals of Periodontology*, Vol.4, #1, Dec. 1999

into subtypes that are either plaque-induced, or related to other systemic influences. Plaque-induced disease may, itself, be modified by systemic factors. Soft Tissue Management[2] is directed at the bacterial component of the disease process.

If the eyes are the windows to the soul, the mouth is the gateway to our health. That's why there is a new understanding of this mouth-body relationship, or what is referred to now as periodontal medicine. We know that bacteria are essential, but insufficient by themselves, to cause disease. There must be a susceptible host. Risk factors for periodontal disease include: genetic predisposition, previous periodontal disease (there is a three-times risk of getting it again), age, gender, medications, diabetes, hormonal change, smoking, poor nutrition, poor oral hygiene, osteoporosis, spousal transmission, clenching/grinding, and stress.

You have the patient with specific bacteria, biologic risk factors, such as systemic diseases, plus genetics and behavioral risk factors, such as poor hygiene, smoking and stress, resulting in a cascade of metabolic changes which, in turn, result in anatomic changes, i.e., bone loss. Patients with periodontitis may have double the risk of developing heart disease. A patient with periodontitis having a heart attack has double the risk of dying from that heart attack!

We've always known that a patient with diabetes is at risk for periodontal disease, but recent studies have shown that patients with periodontal disease have an increased risk of getting diabetes! Hormone replacement therapy may very well be protective from periodontal disease. A patient with periodontal disease is more at risk for respiratory disease and stroke, as well as delivering a premature, low birth-weight baby.

Knowing a patient's risk is necessary to establish an accurate

[2]Soft Tissue Management is a registered trademark of Pro-Dentec, Batesville, AR

diagnosis, treatment plan, maintenance program as well as prognosis. In the "Oral Health in America: A Report of the Surgeon General," June, 2000, the relationship of periodontal disease and systemic disease was confirmed. This has had a dramatic effect on the legal ramifications of early diagnosis, informed consent and early treatment or referral for periodontal disease. There have been reported injury verdicts for the lack of diagnosis and treatment of periodontal disease that are approaching half a million dollars! Diagnosis of periodontal disease is not just about losing teeth anymore!

The goal of Soft Tissue Management is to reduce the bacterial load below the level where there is immune injury, and provide the patient with a structured daily disease control protocol, so as to maximize compliance, and maintain the tissues free of inflammatory changes. The core of this approach to disease management is often the responsibility of the dental hygienist in a general dental office. Once the protocol for treatment has been decided, the hygienist is the principal therapist who implements the program.

The most effective antimicrobial therapy in our armamentarium is the instrumentation of the root surface. Lipopolysaccharide or endotoxin, in the cell wall of the gram-negative anaerobic pathogens, are the initiating causes of periodontal disease. This endotoxin is not deeply embedded in the cemental root surface, as was once believed, but its removal is an essential part of our therapeutic approach. This bacterial component is part of the adherent plaque, which constitutes a destructive biofilm that has been shown to have systemic implications with potentially serious sequelae. Recent studies have shown distinct relationships, as previously discussed, between untreated periodontal disease and serious cardiovascular and pulmonary events.

We have, for many years, recognized the importance of controlling the root surface environment, and have developed various forms of instrumentation to achieve our clinical endpoints in this regard. The addition of ultrasonics in the form of magnetostrictive devices, such as the Cavitron, by Dentsply[3] , took place more than 30 years ago, and was a major step forward. Specifically, these operate at approximately 25-30,000 cycles or vibrations per second, and require a copious amount of water to cool the handpiece and inserts. The tips move in an elliptical pattern requiring multiple, light, overlapping strokes of approximately 50 grams of lateral pressure to detoxify a root surface. The choices from a myriad of tips, and their varied clinical applications, require clinicians to constantly update their knowledge and clinical skills.

More recently, we have developed ultrasonic devices operated by piezoelectric crystals, providing additional levels of efficiency plus patient comfort. Ultrasonic instrumentation, as we know it today, is very technique-sensitive and instrument-specific. There are many manufacturers, and each system has its unique characteristics. The clinician must be familiar with the differences for the best clinical outcome, as well as maximum patient and operator comfort.

Instruments such as the Pro-Select 3[4] , by Pro-Dentec, operate at up to 45,000 cps, providing many more strokes per unit of time than previously available, and at only 3-5 grams of lateral pressure. The three universal tips are effective on all sides, and move in a linear motion that makes access and complete removal of deposits easy and comfortable for the patient. This instrument is a closed system that allows the operator to use a choice of antimicrobials (such as chlorhexidine), as the lavage, instead of water derived from outside

---

[3]Cavitron is a registered trademark of the Dentsply International, York, PA

[4]Pro-Select 3 Piezo Ultrasonic Scaler/Heated Irrigator is a registered trademark of Pro-Dentec, Batesville, AR

sources. Studies have shown that using chlorhexidine as a lavage during ultrasonic instrumentation has a synergistic effect and enhances healing. The Pro-Select 3 is really three systems in one:

> Piezo-ultrasonics, ultrasonics with medicaments and (particularly comfortable for patients), heated subgingival irrigation all through the selection, with a hands-free foot control.

This is the only closed, multi-fluid system available that offers the clinician so many choices for effective instrumentation, also comfort for the patient, as well as providing additional billable services for the practice.

Adjunctive therapy includes additional modalities of both bacterial suppression and modulation of the host immune mechanism. It is used, as the term implies, not as a mono-therapy, or in lieu of basic instrumentation, but to act synergistically with mechanical removal of the biofilm from the root surface to achieve gingival health. Most forms of adjunctive antibacterial therapy involve local or topical delivery systems.

True, legitimate subgingival irrigation, using a cannula to get to the base of the pocket, has mixed reviews in the literature. However, over 60 percent of general dentists provide this as an additional service and part of their Soft Tissue Management programs. With the use of a prescription strength fluoride such as a .63 percent stannous fluoride or a 2 percent neutral sodium fluoride for the suppression of the bacterial rebound and/or to initiate the remineralization process of the root surface following root planing, the hygienist can provide additional services.

The appropriate disease control protocol for the patient at

home would be to apply a maintenance dose of fluoride with a plaque control instrument such as the Rota-dent[5] on a daily basis. Studies have shown that by applying a medicament with the Rota-dent, the rotary action of the fine filaments burnishes the solution into the tooth/soft tissue interface, making the process 30 percent more effective. This assists in the reduction of post-treatment sensitivity, as well as accessing the critical interproximal areas.

Fee ranges for subgingival irrigation range from approximately $12.00 to $40.00 per treatment. Most offices file this service for insurance coverage under the code D9910. Due to synergistic effect, having the patient apply a prescription strength medicine, either a fluoride or chlorhexidine, at home will result in better healing and long-term maintenance. These products, dispensed from the dental office, are filed for insurance benefits under the code D9630. Whether there is insurance coverage or not is unimportant, as patients benefit by reducing the re-formation of plaque, caries protection and control of sensitivity.

Actisite[6], the first of the local drug delivery systems, was introduced about 10 years ago, and proved to be quite effective when used in pockets of 5 mm or more. Actisite is a tetracycline-impregnated fiber that is inserted into the pocket, left for 10 days, then removed. The extremely high concentration of antibiotic results in dramatic reduction of the inflammatory response, and shrinkage of the soft tissue pocket wall. The fiber is always inserted after root planing is completed, as are all the various forms of local or topical drug delivery. Placement of the fiber is tedious, and many times the patient must return within the 10 days for the fiber to be replaced. Cost of this product is about $20 per fiber, and the fees for the placement of this

[5]Rota-dent is a registered trademark of Pro-Dentec, Batesville, AR
[6]Actisite is a registered trademark of Procter & Gamble, Cincinnati, OH

material range from approximately $50 to $150 and are filed under the insurance code D4381.

Two other local delivery systems were introduced in this country in 1998. PerioChip[7] is a concentrated chip of chlorhexidine gluconate which, when inserted in the pocket, slowly biodegrades over a period of one to two weeks, releasing its antibacterial effect over this extended period of time. Placement of the chip is much easier than the fiber; however, one must dry the area extremely well, because if the chip gets wet it does not move into the pocket, but turns into jelly. Letting it warm a little after taking it from the refrigerator allows the clinician to roll the polymer for easier placement into narrow vertical defects or furcations. It is also helpful not to use serrated cotton pliers. These make the chip too difficult to release during placement. Cost of each chip is $14, and the fee range for placement is approximately $35 to $100. It is filed under code D4381.

Atridox[8] is doxycycline delivered in a thixotropic gel. When introduced into the periodontal pocket by means of a dual syringe system, it hardens and remains in place over a one- to two-week period, as it slowly degrades or dissolves. Both of these products are designed to be used in sites unresponsive to traditional scaling and root planing and/or surgery, with residual 5 mm pockets and bleeding upon probing.

Although Atridox is easier to place than the Actisite fiber, there is a learning curve. The gel takes about 30 seconds to begin to harden, then it must be pinched off the end of the cannula by pressing the cannula against the tooth. If this is not done precisely, you will pull it right out of the pocket. Using a wet, small amalgam plugger or plastic instrument to tamp the material into the pocket is helpful.

---

[7]PerioChip is a trademark of Astra Pharmaceuticals, L.P., Westborough, MA
[8]Atridox is a trademark of the Block Drug Corporation, Jersey City, NJ

Completing the procedure by placing a periodontal dressing (as the manufacturer recommends) or using a wet cotton tip to seal the Atridox in the pocket allows the material to stay within the site.

Clinicians have seen some patients with residual amounts of material remaining within the pocket long after two weeks, sometimes creating a mechanical irritant. This is especially true in furcation areas where there may be a mechanical lock of the material. Bringing the patient back for re-evaluation is important. Cost of Atridox is about $52 per syringe system, and the fee range for placement is approximately $100 to $150. This procedure is also filed under code D4381. A narrative such as "because of the unresponsive nature to traditional treatment local antibiotic therapy was necessary" is helpful when submitting to dental insurance.

The decision as to which product you would choose to use in a clinical situation might be based upon: patient's sensitivity to medicament, ease of use or placement, cost factor, number of sites, etc. Many offices choose to use PerioChip if there are one or two sites that require additional treatment, but if there are multiple sites, Atridox is used since the syringe system contains enough material for up to three or four sites.

A review article by Dr. Gary Greenstein, "The Role of Local Drug Delivery in the Management of Periodontal Diseases: A Comprehensive Review," published in *J. Periodontal*, May 1998, states there is no universally superior system at this time.

There are other similar controlled delivery systems in use, but not yet available in the United States. All of these adjunctive modalities have been shown to concentrate their antibacterial activity in the pocket, where they are needed, with barely measurable amounts found in the systemic circulation. They all result in some pocket reduction via shrinkage of the soft tissue wall, and some slight (average .3 mm) gain in clinical attachment level.

The adjunctive therapy systems outlined above are all aimed at controlling the bacterial component of the disease process. We know the host immune response represents the other side of the equation, resulting in pathology. Considerable research, therefore, has been directed at developing approaches that provide us the ability to modulate the cascade of events that result in attachment loss or disease activity.

The tetracycline family of antibiotics possesses a unique corollary effect in addition to their bacteriostatic ability. They inhibit the formation of collagenase, an enzyme that degrades the integrity of the connective tissue and bony matrix, resulting in attachment loss. This effect is independent of any antibacterial action.

Periostat[9], introduced in 1998, is a 20 mg tablet of doxycycline hyclate. When taken twice daily it has absolutely no antibacterial effect, but stops the collagenolytic action of disease activity. It is therefore, the first form of therapy aimed at modulating the host immune response, and is used in conjunction with root instrumentation, as an adjunctive therapy. A prescription may be for the time during active therapy, and continued for up to nine months. Compliance by the patient is always an issue, as well as the cost factor. However, studies have shown, and it has been anecdotally seen, that this enhances the clinical results of traditional mechanical therapy.

The hygiene department can significantly impact not only patient care, but the bottom line of the practice, by diversifying services. Home bleaching systems are a way that dentistry can provide what our patients really want--whiter, more attractive teeth! There are a number of home bleaching systems available on the market. Most of

---

[9]Periostat is a registered trademark of the CollaGenex Pharmaceutical, Cherry Hill, NJ

the products contain carbamide peroxide in varying percentages. Using a custom tray made within the dental office provides a vehicle to carry and hold the bleaching gel against the tooth. The strength and viscosity of the material, as well as contact time, determines the results.

A few professional products contain a combination of hydrogen peroxide and carbamide peroxide. Tooth and soft tissue sensitivity are a concern, and some kits include neutral sodium fluoride gels. Office observations and monitoring are essential for the best results and patient satisfaction. Having a system within the office for discussing the patient's desires as well as expectations is critical for patient satisfaction. There are, of course, in-office whitening systems, some using white lights, while others use lasers. Dental boards are establishing guidelines as to the role of the dental team with these types of bleaching systems.

Unfortunately, there are more and more products for whitening, as well as other procedures, available over-the-counter that could be harmful to patients. The dental professional must take an active role in discussing all over-the-counter dental procedures as regards appropriateness, safety and efficacy.

Note from Dr. Wilde:
As I have stated in previous chapters, Soft Tissue Management is what made my hygiene department successful and I have asked Jane Jones to describe how to get this program structured in your practice. Jane contributed to the development of the original Soft Tissue Management curriculum by Pro-Dentec, the company that structured and "packaged" this concept. She has lectured extensively in the US and Canada on the subject and is a known authority in the conversion of "cleaning departments" to profitable "perio-hygiene departments." If your hygiene production isn't in the range of $2-300,000 annually, read on.

ADDENDUM

An ACTION PLAN for PROFITABLE DENTAL HYGIENE

It is by design that this ADDENDUM is in the middle of Dr. Wilde's book. The first half shows readers why hygiene should be profitable, with examples of his success. The second half shows doctors the benefits of a profitable hygiene department and how to experience financial freedom. Where I come in is to reassure all the readers that they are not alone in questions such as, Whom do I turn to for step-by-step implementation? Where do I start? How do I get my team going? Where do I go (grow) from here? The answers lie within these pages. How to:

- **Structure an organized SYSTEM for perio**
- **Get your entire team on the same page**
- **Acquire tools that communicate treatment VALUE to patients**
- **Get Soft Tissue Management going and measure the growth**
- **Present treatment to patients with confidence**
- **Create comfortable, successful treatment strategies**

Stephen Covey advises in his book, *The Seven Habits of Highly Effective People*, **"Begin with the end in mind." Dr. Wilde summarizes in his Conclusion with three primary themes:** ***Value Clarification, Systems Refinement,*** and ***Wisdom occurs when Action is taken*****. Here's where we need to begin, the VALUE question.**

Why do dental offices provide periodontal therapy for prophy fees? It begins in hygiene school. For years dental hygiene

students are taught optimum patient care: Always put the needs of the patient first. What a great foundation on which dental hygiene education is based and is still taught today! However, in most academic situations, these hygiene (and dental) programs teach the necessary skills for optimum patient care but the fee that is charged to the clinic patient is whatever that institution deems appropriate. Most of the time it is barely enough to cover the supplies used in that patient care. Because profitability is not an issue, new graduates have no sense of *VALUE* in their services from a monetary or business perspective. When new graduates leave academia and enter the "real world," they are not only faced with a schedule of 8 or more patients per day (as compared to having 1 patient all year in school), but now, there is a fee associated with those patients. Hopefully, those fees are commensurate with the value of the services.

The problem compounds itself when a new graduate enters an office with an existing staff that has always "done it that way" and cannot teach this new "dentling" the real world. Is it any wonder that the hygiene department is a frustrating financial drain on the practice as opposed to being a profitable dental hygiene department?

As hygienists, some years back, we were also taught that calculus was the cause of periodontal disease and we were evaluated in school as well as on our state boards by our ability to remove calculus. Is it any wonder that calculus and stain removal were our primary focus? The scene is set, we have existing patients who want to have their teeth "cleaned," a hygiene department that is schedule-driven and hygienists who want to do meticulous work. Doing prophys, however, in a pool of blood with the patient com-

ing back in 6 months so we can do it all over again is very frustrating! Is this, also, supervised neglect?

Beginning in the mid-1980s a paradigm shift started to happen. There was new research and information regarding periodontal disease. General dental practices started facing their fears to diagnose, treat and charge for nonsurgical periodontal services, and, at the same time, Pro-Dentec®, Inc., emerged as a new company. Dr. Wilde gives credit to Pro-Dentec as the source of information through its Soft Tissue Management® seminars, support services and quality products that, literally, transformed his hygiene department. ***Finally, the VALUE of the hygiene department was realized!***

Pro-Dentec was started by businessmen and has grown to include general dentists, periodontists, orthodontists, endodontists, hygienists, assistants, business management, and insurance personnel. In other words, they are a huge dental team. Their initial goal was to provide a quality educational and training service to dentists and hygienists who were recommending Rota-dent® for patient plaque control at home. Little did they know that this idea would actually evolve into the program called Soft Tissue Management. In 1985 if you asked a group of general dentists how many were diagnosing and treating early-stage periodontal disease, only a few hands (if any) would go up. There was a tremendous void between a prophylaxis and flap surgery. Pro-Dentec recognized the dental profession needed a structured approach to nonsurgical periodontal therapy, and in 1985 actually created the term and system called Soft Tissue Management.

Pro-Dentec can take much of the credit for the change in emphasis by general dentists to provide nonsurgical periodontal

treatment for their patients. How did they do that? Interestingly enough, they decided to go into partnership with the dental profession. Their products are only available through dental offices, so helping the profession is definitely in their best interest.

Mission Statement

Pro-Dentec is dedicated to designing and manufacturing innovative products and disseminating information to dental professionals for the diagnosis, treatment and prevention of periodontal and other diseases.

We are committed to elevating the standard of care in the dental industry by providing technology supporting excellence in dentistry.

Pro-Dentec's commitment to clinical excellence evolved into continuing education seminars for the entire dental team for a nominal tuition. The value is that everyone is on the same page and understands the Soft Tissue Management System. Their STM seminar outlines the role of each team member in how to implement a structured system of early diagnosis and early treatment of periodontal disease including the maintenance phase of patient care. Special emphasis is on behavior modification in the patient which is mandatory to the success of treatment as described as follows by the American Dental Association in their Risk Management Series.

"In viewing periodontal treatment, the role of the patient should not be overlooked. The patient must be an active participant in the treatment through compliance, in fact, the role of the patient is paramount to the success of therapy."

Pro-Dentec's commitment to customer service is embodied in hundreds of employees, many of whom work within these dental teams as extended team members. They provide personalized services as the offices go through the process of implementing Soft Tissue Management, and this commitment is time-tested and unique. Their dedication to quality is an ongoing pursuit to manufacture products that are directly related to helping the dental practices provide the highest quality of care in their hygiene departments. It is this enhanced quality of care that is the cornerstone of increased production and profits from hygiene with existing patients.

Once you are a customer of Pro-Dentec's, there is a plethora of ongoing personalized literature and patient education materials that assist the dental team in communicating the value of treatment versus a routine cleaning. The patient education aids, personalization and marketing materials are designed to keep patients in the dental office, coming back for additional services. The principles and ethics of Pro-Dentec begin with the owners and are shared among its people. From the beginning, they have been involved with cancer research and are committed to donate a portion of the sales proceeds of all their products toward the goal of finding a cure for cancer and providing scholarships for those people who need assistance in seeking care.

SYSTEMS REFINEMENT is Dr. Wilde's second theme throughout this book. **Having a system that is a structured, organ-**

ized Soft Tissue Management Program is the basic foundation from which not only is quality patient care delivered but hygiene production triples! It involves the entire team! STM is a system starting with the patient's first phone call, and covers how they are greeted at the office, the co-examination process, patient education, optimum periodontal therapy, personalized behavior modification, individualized maintenance program and/or a referral protocol.

Thousands of offices around the country have implemented Pro-Dentec's Soft Tissue Management Program. They not only have experienced the professional satisfaction of doing the right thing for the patient but have enjoyed the obvious benefits of increased hygiene production as well as an increase in restorative production. When the patients feel in control, their mouths feel, taste and smell better; they literally partner with the dental office. The dental office they once feared. The improved relationship leads to higher case acceptance of the restorative or cosmetic treatment plan and new patient referrals as well. There is also less patient "fallout." Recall retention increases, which translates directly to the bottom line.

How does all this happen? Thousands of offices have attended the Soft Tissue Management Seminars, sponsored by Pro-Dentec, and continue to do so on a yearly basis. The seminars are presented by practicing dentists who actually teach what has become the standard of care for treating periodontal disease. The entire dental team is encouraged to attend because everyone has a role. The front office staff is coached on handling the patient's first phone call into the practice as well as how to use the patient questionnaire that begins the co-diagnosis process. A thorough review of the patient's medical history is even more important

than ever with the evidence linking periodontal disease to systemic diseases. A discussion of the patient's medications as well as nutritional supplements, especially herbals, is included in this patient assessment of risk for periodontal disease.

Periodontal disease is epidemic! It is second only to the common cold. It is the No. 1 reason for tooth loss in adults! However, with early diagnosis and treatment it is controllable. To assist in this educational process, Pro-Dentec provides personalized brochures as well as scripts for the dental team. This sequence of events leads the patient into the co-examination process.

Just as we use an explorer to determine if the patient has decay or defective restorations, we use a periodontal probe to determine the health of the gums. "When the probe appears, the disease appears." That statement is the basis of a Soft Tissue Management Program. Following the American Dental Association's guidelines since the middle 1980s, offices must perform a full mouth probing at least on an annual basis to determine the periodontal status of their patients and their stability during maintenance.

A structured system and the time involved are two reasons why patients are not routinely probed and charted. Again, Pro-Dentec has addressed this concern by manufacturing a pressure-sensitive probe, the Sensor™ Probe, which helps dentists and hygienists to standardize and calibrate their techniques. A new system now available from Pro-Dentec, the STM Probe™ is a battery-operated, automated, pressure-sensitive probe. The STM Probe does not require a foot control since all feedback is through the handpiece itself. The comfortable disposable tips are attached to a handpiece that registers the components of a periodontal eval-

uation with audible feedback so that the clinician can perform the evaluation working alone. When patients hear their "numbers" with a summary of their periodontal evaluation printed out for them, there is no question about case acceptance.

For those offices that are hesitant to start STM because of the time it takes to perform the periodontal evaluation, here's the answer. The hygienists can now collect the data by themselves in less than 10 minutes! This is critical documentation for medical/legal reasons, also. With all the new information linking periodontal disease with systemic diseases, it's not just about the teeth anymore. Legal settlements for the lack of diagnosis and treatment of periodontal disease have now escalated from $10,000 per tooth to jury verdicts of over $498,000!

Once the doctor makes the diagnosis the patient is presented a treatment plan specifically designed for his or her level of disease. These treatment plans have been previously thought out by the dental team and printed out as a "blueprint" for the appropriate treatment for each patient. This "blueprint" is the first key to success for Soft Tissue Management. Just as Dr. Wilde described his treatment plans in a previous chapter, the dental practices that partner with Pro-Dentec are provided comfortable, successful treatment strategies for each level of periodontal disease including localized disease. These treatment plans reflect:

- **the number of appointments necessary**
- **the services that are to be rendered at each appointment**
- **the length of each appointment**
- **the interval between appointments**
- **the total fee for both the in-office and the home care treatment**

This structure, which is described in detail in Pro-Dentec's STM seminars, is personalized for each office during a follow-up staff meeting facilitated by a highly trained professional representative from the company. The entire dental team is assisted with scheduling, current insurance codes and narratives. How to utilize personalized patient education and in-office training materials is a part of the services as well as role-playing communication skills for optimum case acceptance. In case presentation, quoting one fee for the entire treatment, both in-office as well as coordinated home treatment, is the second key to success for Soft Tissue Management.

These professional representatives are also trained in staff development and motivation techniques and are committed to assist the doctor in working with his/her dental team. These services are complimentary to valued clients of Pro-Dentec. They not only equal, but exceed those of some highly paid consultants that see you for a designated time and then periodically give you a phone call. These representatives and the ongoing training by Pro-Dentec fill a unique marketing niche, exclusively providing products and services as a partner with the dental profession!

We now know more about the nature and etiology of periodontal disease. This knowledge combined with new technology has changed the way we treat our patients. This not only challenges us to update our clinical skills but to re-evaluate the equipment needed to deliver optimum care. Again, Pro-Dentec, after reviewing the current research and working with professional focus groups, designed and manufactures the latest technology in the nonsurgical treatment of periodontal disease, the Pro-Select 3™ Piezo-Ultrasonic Scaler with heated subgingival irrigation. It is truly a one-of-kind periodontal therapy system! Patients are

more comfortable during treatment with a reduced need for anesthesia, hygienists are more comfortable and confident in delivering meticulous treatment, and additional billable services are provided with this periodontal therapy system.

Studies have shown that ultrasonic instrumentation is equal to hand instruments but faster. Not all ultrasonics are the same, however. Older technology causes patient discomfort and is cumbersome for hygienists to operate. The Pro-Select 3 handpiece is very lightweight and the 45,000 linear vibrations per second of the ultra-thin tips result in a gentle "no hammering" effect unlike that which patients have experienced with other powered scalers. Three reservoirs provide the clinician a choice of medicaments to use, such as an antimicrobial or a desensitizing fluoride, while scaling and root planing. This allows the hygienist to keep the patient more comfortable and greatly reduces the need for anesthesia.

Instead of performing one quadrant of root planing per visit, many offices with the Pro-Select 3 schedule patients with moderate periodontal disease for an extended appointment and treat two quadrants. This is a tremendous benefit to the patients because time is such an issue. The benefit to the practice is that patients may be comfortably scheduled for root planing back to back. The Pro-Select 3 Piezo-Ultrasonic Scaler/Irrigator is ranked No. 1 by a nationally recognized independent research group.

Recognized authorities in the area of periodontics believe that the treatment of periodontal disease is 30 percent clinical and 70 percent behavioral. Studies also show that the fewer things we ask patients to do on a daily basis, the more likely they are to do them. Compliance is key to the success in treating periodontal disease. University-based studies on the Rota-dent prove that for

interproximal access there is no comparable power or manual brush. Periodontal disease is an interproximal disease. We know that it starts and is more severe in between the teeth. Combining home care with the in-office treatment gives the clinician and the patient the control necessary to arrest the disease and maintain the health and stability achieved through active therapy.

It has been shown through a 10-year study that patients who use the Rota-dent vs. those using manual methods for plaque control were more effective in their daily care but, more importantly, were dedicated to 3-month maintenance intervals to the level of 92 percent! What does that mean to the dental practice? Patients not only achieve better dental health, but, because of the relationship between the patient and the practice, they return for care and refer others to the office. Including the Rota-dent as part of the total treatment and fee communicates to the patient that home care needs are not optional and are the third key to success for Soft Tissue Management. Providing a professional solution to make the patient's all-important role of daily plaque control easier and more effective results in treatment success.

Three Keys to Success

Printed blueprints for each case type

One fee for the in-office and home treatment

Behavior modification with Rota-dent

The commitment by Pro-Dentec to keep the Rota-dent in the dental office actually came as a request of the dental profession. Those involved with the numerous studies on the Rota-dent said that the best approach for patients is to receive personalized instructions on their daily plaque control. Retail products which have misleading "Wall Street advertising" claims are not the best value for our patient's dental dollars. Pro-Dentec is a dedicated partner with the dental profession to help provide the patient with the best possible care, to support and help train the staff, facilitate the increase in production, and establish monitoring systems so that the doctor's net increases. Does it get any better than that?

SYSTEMS REFINEMENT **is what this is all about. It's the No. 1 reason why dental teams attend Pro-Dentec's STM seminars, and that's what they get!** ***SYSTEM*** **could be an acronym for S̲ave Y̲ou S̲tress, T̲ime, E̲ffort and M̲oney. Pro-Dentec delivers that System, as taught in the seminars and implemented with the help of highly trained professional representatives supported by their products, services and people who have made a difference in dentistry.**

WISDOM OCCURS WHEN ACTION IS TAKEN. **This is Dr. Wilde's third theme in his summary. All the best intentions do not happen until action is taken. What is your next step? Make two simple commitments, but, remember, a commitment is not a decision, it is an** ***Action*****!**

1. Commit to probe and chart every patient!
2. Call Pro-Dentec, 1-800-228-5595

Let's face it. No matter what stage of Soft Tissue Management you have implemented, wouldn't it be prudent to partner with Pro-Dentec to ***Save You Stress, Time, Effort and Money*****?**

SEGMENT II

TECHNIQUES TO ENHANCE PATIENT VOLUME

Chapter 6

Beginning Expanded Hygiene and Marketing Basics

As far as I'm concerned, you can quit reading right now. Most everything I know, and all the information that it is essential to comprehend to enable one to establish a dynamic, highly effective and profitable hygiene department has been covered. At the very least, there is no reason to put off getting started on your journey to obtain all the benefits accompanying profitable dental hygiene I've described. But precisely how does one begin?

The first step is to carefully consider one's current position. If you already have the available space and hygienist, begin to discuss this information with your hygienist, and together, formulate a plan leading to a brighter future for dentist, hygienist, staff and patients. You need only be sure that all parties have a firm grasp of the logistics we've already discussed (i.e., understand how expanded hygiene functions), settle the compensation issue, hire a hygiene assistant and begin to gear up scheduling for increased profitability.

If all that delays you is adding a hygiene assistant, as previously mentioned, I've updated our hiring system from *Bringing Your Practice Into Focus*, and placed it in the appendix. It seems in most books, material relegated to the appendix is not worth reading. I've delegated our hiring information to the book's end, as it doesn't directly relate to hygiene. **But the hiring information I've included--though admittedly not critical for adding a hygienist--is ideal for all other team positions, and is easily worth the investment you've made in the book**! Nothing is more essential to success than surrounding yourself with the right team. Nothing destroys the heart of a practice, or the soul of a dentist, more certainly than being forced to work with people who don't share one's values, dreams and visions.

The painstaking, detailed system our practice uses to identify ideal team members requires a lot of effort, but it has been tested and refined for over 20 years in our office. When carefully and thoughtfully implemented, it allows one almost unbelievable insight into the true character of potential employees. Can one pick and choose portions of the system to implement? Be my guest, but don't expect similar results from diminished efforts. I hope this doesn't come as a shock, but the world doesn't work that way.

Yes, the system is time-consuming, but the investment required to find the perfect employee is minuscule compared to the heartache and waste involved with hiring wrong, suffering with that individual through a period of training, than admitting your mistake and having to start the search all over again.

If you need a hygienist (or an additional one), the obvious place to begin is with the recruitment material just covered. I understand that it's hard to find hygienists, but if you employ all the techniques I've described, as diligently as possible, you'll be successful in your quest. The key is **massive action**...begin all efforts at once, bringing to bear all the power you can muster, to maximize recruiting results.

Before you bring in a hygienist candidate to interview, be sure you've created a work space that looks and is equipped in a manner consistent with your clear values and the top-quality staff member you wish to employ. Remember, you may only get one shot at hiring your ideal person. Don't describe your plans for the future, but create the ideal space you've envisioned in which he or she can perform, and have it waiting.

By having this optimal environment prepared in advance, you'll show applicants you are truly committed, not just dreaming. If you think, "But, wouldn't it be safer to wait until I've hired someone?", review my profit history again. Such achievements aren't accomplished by those with weak wills, or who hesitate to commit and act decisively. The highest levels of achievement, in all fields, are reserved for those with clear visions and unwavering determination. A lot of excellent offices desire the finest hygienists. The day--and the ideal team member--belongs to the bold.

It's possible the problem you must overcome concerns your facility. (If you wish to grow, it's a given there will be problems to surmount, no matter what the issue in question! Let me hasten to point out this reality is NOT my idea!) Perhaps you have the space available, and only need to add equipment, and find creative ways to schedule to make expanded hygiene a reality.

Maybe you need to remodel your office to accommodate another hygiene room. I believe an office that speaks of excellence needs to be remodeled about every five years anyway. I don't mean touching up the paint, but carpet, wallcovering, artwork, possibly furniture, even walls changed.

You and your staff deserve a lovely new environment more than the patients, if for no other reason than the sheer weight of the hours you spend there. It's been my experience that such improvements fire everyone up, and quickly pay for themselves through the enhanced productivity that accompanies such excitement. Considering the potential profits we've discussed, a remodeling job should not present a great obstacle to anyone who is sincere in his or her desires to become more.

It's time for dentistry to embrace the fact that **WE RUN A BUSINESS**, and begin to function in a rational, businesslike manner. Making the accommodations required for something as profitable as expanded hygiene is hardly a tough financial call! Once again, compare, with your newly acquired understanding, your past hygiene profit results to my averages. The additional profit accruing from one month of fully functioning expanded hygiene can pay for a great deal of refurbishing.

And maybe studying this tome will mark one of the great moments of passage in your career. You may determine that NOW is the time to move to a facility where you can achieve the practice of your dreams. (If this is the case, chances are you already knew it at some level of awareness...but perhaps needed a nudge to move into action.) Honestly consider if the office in which you now work makes it possible to achieve the desires of your professional future. If the answer is clearly NO, and I've forced you to that cliff...I hope you jump. Life is too short, too precious, not to try to be as fulfilled as possible.

A new office represents a major commitment of time, energy and financial resources. Work the numbers, enlisting the help of an accountant, if necessary. Whether to relocate or stay put is determined by financial projections of future revenue and profits, not by one's emotions of the moment.

Certainly there exists an ideal physical resource for the unique practice each dentist envisions, but I'm horrified to read of offices that win those awards for "practice of the year," often sponsored by equipment companies. If they want me to study that "information," they'll have to start including a profit and loss statement, along with all the pretty pictures. It doesn't take much intelligence, skill or insight to buy every piece of equipment ever made, and hang it on the dang wall. Have these people ever heard of overhead? Almost any dentist can borrow money. It's the paying back that presents a challenge.

A pleasant, warm, professional office that **functions ideally** is all any dentist needs. Waste your money, if you must splurge, on staff. It's the people, not the equipment, that determine how well any practice will do. One of my heroes, and the creative inspiration for a generation (or two), of dentists, Dr. Earl Estep, calls offices with the marble columns and indoor swimming pools "monuments to the dentist's ego." There exist much cheaper, more efficient ways to deal with self-esteem problems. (Even at $10 per tablet, Viagra is a lot chcaper than a new office. So is buying a sports car, if your knees still allow ingress and egress....I'm determined to ignore the symbolism of my beloved 12-gauge Browning shotguns.)

Whatever the logistical challenge one must overcome, get after it. Relatively concrete and predictable solutions can be developed to deal with any of the above discussed problems. The following information, some of which originally appeared in Chapter 3 of *Dentistry's Future*, is to assist those who need more patient volume to fully schedule expanded hygiene.

Even if you lack sufficient patients to begin full-time expanded hygiene at the moment, consider condensing hygiene days and going expanded on a part-time basis. Such a business decision will increase your profit, enhance hygienist compensation and attitude, and allow additional time to be available for each patient. (There is also a wonderful bonus possible with part-time expanded--days with no hygiene checks--ideal for large cases, high production and reduced stress.)

Again, I include the following completely rewritten material to make this book a stand-alone resource, although I must warn you, once expanded hygiene is up and going, you'll probably realize you need an associate, and have to purchase *Dentistry's Future* to discover the secrets of small group practices anyway. That book does for group practice what this book does for hygiene...moves it into the future.

As some of the already shared statistics from my practice indicated (consider my $6,000-plus per-day NET average), a well run group practice that includes a profitable hygiene system can be much more lucrative than any solo endeavor, while allowing the owner-dentist greater freedom.

Increasing New Patient Volume

It seems every dentist--no matter how busy or successful--thinks he needs more new patients, and in our current economy of high incomes, low unemployment, and a steadily decreasing supply of dentists, getting them is not a big challenge, if one has a fully functional new-patient recruitment SYSTEM perpetually in place.

No matter how many loyal patients one's practice enjoys, it's usually true that the highest quality of care one delivers, and often the most profitable, is derived from new clients. Typically, new patients tend to be highly motivated to solve whatever oral health concerns they perceived themselves to have, which led them to schedule an examination appointment.

But a lot of "dental marketing" leaves us uneasy, as it violates our values. I believe all but those of you too busy to see even one more patient will enjoy the following down-to-earth, ethically comfortable marketing information.

Here's a basic fact that often seems to be overlooked. The ultimate reason patients come to, then stay with a dental practice is that they believe this dentist and office can be trusted to provide the best possible care consistent with their personal values and interests. This is true of the poor soul who just wants an aching molar removed, as well as the 24-veneer case of your most demanding and refined patient.

DO WHAT YOU MUST TO BECOME THAT TRUSTED PERSON BY CONSISTENTLY ACTING IN A MANNER CONSISTENT WITH YOUR EMPHATICALLY CLARIFIED VALUES!!

There is nothing wrong with making efforts to identify oneself to others as the dentist they seek (marketing). But any accomplishment less than achieving a thorough understanding of human nature, and always trying to do one's best for another, will eventually lead to professional disaster, no matter how massive the hordes of patients attracted to one's practice by the most skilled and sophisticated marketing.

If an office can't deliver what their marketing message promises, patients will soon discover this discrepancy and feel deceived and betrayed. They will probably leave angrily, telling others of their negative experience and disappointment. I believe this is as it should be...both just and fair. **For a marketing plan to ultimately succeed, its message must accurately reflect the practice as it exists.**

This general caveat in place, let's consider my personal philosophy, and the techniques by which we assist patients in discovering our office is the perfect place for them to receive their dental care.

I'll remain candid. For the majority of my career, I didn't display much interest or expertise concerning the overt or external marketing of my practice. True, I've always marketed internally, by working hard to please each patient and giving more than expected, I hope in a behaviorally adept manner.

But, as I added associates and reduced my hours in the office, I marketed a little more each year. As I do with every endeavor, once committed to deliberate patient recruitment, I became a student, attending courses and reading books on the subject.

The reason I never marketed as a solo dentist was because I was always too busy to handle the farrago of patients who wandered in, almost from the day I first opened the office doors. The precise historic details are a bit obscure (I didn't get much sleep in those days, and had not developed the office monitors we've briefly discussed), but for approximately four years, our office did not accept new patients, as we were booked three or more months in advance. (The pressure of constantly working patients into the schedule, starting early and always finishing late, about killed me, and that--not enhanced net--was my major motivation for seeking an associate dentist to HELP!)

The gurus of the industry might suggest I was scheduled months in advance because of inefficiencies that "clogged my schedule." I would counter that I suffered from the effort to provide the best dental care I possibly could to over 5,000 very active patients...a staggering, impossible load!

Before adding an associate, I did everything in my power to accommodate patient demand and maximize productivity. I had five fully equipped operatories, a staff of seven, had implemented expanded hygiene, studied books and magazines, timed every clinical procedure (see Chapter 12 of *Focus* for specifics concerning the vital task of constructing a **scheduling ruler**, a simple idea that contains amazing power to enhance efficiency, productivity and profit), took numerous courses and hired consultants to help streamline every office system.

I was producing $40,000 per month as a solo dentist around 1982--when that was a relatively significant amount of money.

(Assuming 4 percent inflation during this 18-year interval, this would equate to approximately $81,000 per month in today's weakened dollars. I know...it's still weak beer to many of the profession's heavy hitters. I'm just telling you what I've done.)

My office overhead had gradually drifted toward 70 percent, as patient overload left little time for organization, and inefficiency was compounded by fatigue. When we added an associate, and I began to reduce chairside hours to allow myself more time to manage, practice overhead dropped to around 50 percent, where it has generally remained. (The increased production/ increased net/ decreased overhead of a multi-dentist practice is the primary triple-booster rocket to net income, and explaining how to create such a system was the main reason I wrote *Dentistry's Future*.)

Attracting patients in abundance is a critical portion of practice success. Marketing is one possible method whereby one may achieve this goal, especially helpful during the early years of a practice, or when implementing significant enhancements--such as adding expanded hygiene or an associate dentist--all situations when a robust flow of new patients is acutely needed.

Once again, I've shared my personal experience to explain the context from which I present marketing data, thus enabling this information to be more thoroughly and honestly interpreted. The history lesson completed for now, let's return our focus to patient recruitment.

Everyone Markets

Marketing encompasses every interaction any member of an office team has with another person. You "market" when you smile and nod to someone on the street, as well as when launching a $10,000 television advertising venture. (TV marketing is something I've never even considered. Another step on the long journey of subjects about which I know nothing.)

Staff members market when visiting with a neighbor they happen to meet in the grocery store. Marketing includes views--good and bad--shared about one's office over the fence (where Iowa neighbors often converse during pleasant weather) or over the phone. In its broadest context, marketing is the way one presents himself or herself-clothes, speech, walk, behavior, etc.--in one's efforts to gain acceptance, and avoid rejection, by other community members.

(In ancient tribal communities, banishment from society was a sentence of death, except perhaps for Tarzan. Subliminal memories of this reality might explain why the pain of rejection is more piquant than would seem logical.)

So, dentist or non-dentist, no one can avoid marketing. (In the final analysis, irrespective of occupation or motivation, all one has to sell is himself or herself.) One can choose to market with awareness and purpose, in a manner consistent with thoughtfully defined personal values, or stumble along, without clear direction, hoping everything somehow works out for the best.

(Take a moment and consider which approach you have been employing. How's it working to date? It might help further refine the premise to consider tongue-piercing as a form of marketing message, although glossal perforation--except as an indication of intelligence quotient--is one signal the meaning of which I fear I'm too old to grasp. I think I'm glad about that.) Allow me to share my personal definition of dental marketing...one unlike any I've seen in print:

Professional marketing includes any manner of displaying one's beliefs and values to the public, thus to position one's business by defining to others WHAT ONE BELIEVES IN, thereby attracting consumers with similar interests and opinions. Please contemplate this statement carefully. As we proceed, evaluate each topic considered as it relates to this standard. I think one will discover this definition describes and encompasses every effective marketing activity we'll consider. Problems arise when one's values aren't clear, and thus the marketing message--in its varied forms--is changeable, muddled, sporadic and confusing.

I'll take no chance that this crucial, pivotal premise can be misunderstood. The most critical segment of an effective marketing plan is the pristine definition of beliefs and values by the dental office leader--YOU, DOCTOR. This clear vision creates consistency, thus power.

While form will vary substantially, based on unique beliefs and circumstances, here are the primary ingredients of every successful marketing concept:

1. Values are precisely articulated, then coalesced into written form by a unified dental team. This is the critical first step--the clarified statement of why an office exists--that creates the foundation upon which all success rests. This may be codified in the form of a document often described as the office purpose, or mission statement.

   Our office mission statement, over a year in completion, is as follows:

   Our office exists to serve the people we have dedicated ourselves to...our patients. We will create an environment of honesty and professionalism where patients will feel comfortable, cared for, and welcome. All patients will be aware of the quality of care they receive, and the sincere care of the staff for them.

   We pledge to be positive, supportive team members, and to create a place where we are able to have fun, while encouraging and supporting personal and professional growth.

2. Clear values, combined with energy and some creative thought (aided, perhaps, by some external stimulation, as from an excellent course, newsletter or magazine article, or say...an exciting dental book!) lead to developing an advertising scheme that defines one's mission to the public. This concise expression of office beliefs and benefits serves to attract patients, especially people with values similar to those of the practice. (And life is so much more enjoyable when spent in the company of those with similar values, be they patients, staff, or family and loved ones.)

3. IT IS CRITICAL THAT THE MESSAGE OF EVERY FORM OF ADVERTISING--from the hello and smile to a neighbor in the store, to the quality of the practice stationery, to the reception-room reading materials, to the expensive television campaign--be **invariably, perfectly aligned in every nuance, with these carefully defined values**.

4. To be effective, a marketing message must also be **consistently REPEATED**--not just reactivated when "things are slow" in the office.

   Erratic marketing efforts were the norm in our practice for years. Campaigns were mounted when increased new-patient flow was required (usually when a full-time associate was added), then abandoned when we got too busy, only to be laboriously resurrected years later when we again needed more patients. We kept reinventing and re-implementing similar marketing strategies, and these concepts required time, money and energy to employ and achieve results, on every occasion in which we resurrected them.

We ended this ineptness by designating one staff member as our permanent public relations leader, and having her create a monthly calendar of PR events that we follow throughout the year. We review, discuss and evaluate each month's plans, and assign specific PR tasks to team members, during our regular monthly staff meetings.

(A sample of our PR calendar is located at the end of Segment II.)

Developing an Effective Game Plan

I hope non-basketball fans will indulge me for falling back on an old passion to illustrate a point. A great coach (practice leader) will assess his or her basketball team (dental staff) and define what it is they do best, and in what areas they are deficient.

Perhaps the coach discovers his or her team is quick, has good depth, is composed of excellent athletes, but ones of small stature. This analysis carefully completed--because upon its accuracy the team will succeed or fail--a scheme is developed to optimize their unique blend of talents.

A quick, small athletic team might be best suited to play a full-court, pressing defense the entire game, thus employing their strengths to harass larger, more powerful teams into mistakes and turnovers that lead to easy baskets.

The same coach, working with a big team in another season, may wish to fall back on defense, and slowly walk the ball up the floor, then work the ball inside, near the basket, to take advantage of players size and "pound the boards" for rebounds.

Whatever the scheme developed, every member of the organization must understand and enthusiastically support their portion of the plan. The strategy must be consistently practiced and constantly employed for the team to achieve the greatest possible success of which it is capable. Any deviation from this ideal course must be immediately identified and corrected.

As one begins to clarify one's values, the key question to be answered is, what is your ideal dental scheme? (Marketing is merely a single--if highly visible--facet of one's office values and identity.) Does the dentist wear a silk tie, the office play soothing baroque music and feature *Barron's* and *The Wall Street Journal* as reading materials in the reception area?

Or does the dress code consist of designer jeans, the music rock and roll, and does the reception room feature *People* magazine? **BOTH STYLES, AND ALL IN BETWEEN, CAN BE EFFECTIVE, IF CAREFULLY DESIGNED TO MAXIMIZE TEAM STRENGTHS, AND CONSISTENTLY PORTRAYED**. But when a big team tries to fast-break, or a "Wall Street Journal" office goes to jeans, identity has been lost, and trouble soon ensues. Mixed messages confuse, and it is impossible to market effectively when you have not precisely defined what you are selling.

To summarize, lucid practice visions begin with the dentist taking whatever time is required to envision the office of his or her dreams. This revelation is repeatedly explained, refined and enhanced at every opportunity, to anyone who will listen. When office beliefs are clear and compelling to all team members, consistency in marketing, and every other facet of office appearance and behavior, will not present a problem. If precise goals are unclear, and thus preferred behavior uncertain, office policy will change with every meeting attended, every book read...and chaos results.

Characteristics of the John Wilde Marketing Program

Let's examine the universal or generic characteristics of what I consider to be an effective dental marketing strategy, before discussing my specific techniques and programs.

1. **Professional**--To me this means a marketing strategy:

   a) To which I am proud to have my name attached. (I believe each of the examples that follow will support and illustrate this contention--although a precise definition of professionalism will vary, profoundly influenced by individual situations, values and taste.)

   b) The focus of every message is on service to the public through dental health education.

   c) Each message must enhance the strength of the entire dental profession. If one falls prey to an overt self-focus--for example, by trumpeting self-proclaimed (and self-perceived) personal superiority over other dental health-care providers--such self-interest becomes apparent, and results in decreased trust, at least among discerning people. (The need to be perceived as "better" than others is a certain sign of self-esteem problems. Take it from someone who has battled such painful insecurity for a lifetime.)

2. **Inexpensive**--I'm cheap. I also am concerned with enhancing my profit through marketing, not just "positioning my office," or making a name for myself in the community. (If one's goal is simply to become well known in the community, get busted for drugs, hookers, or other "front page" topics. Folks will become aware of you, almost instantly!)

   I dislike using marketing programs where I can't measure results, and where the money allocated is not quickly returned multiple times. I consider marketing an investment, and as with any business venture, one should be able to measure results, and expect to demonstrate a clear profit.

3. **FUN**--Every activity employed to promote the practice must be enjoyable for both patients and staff. Our team (okay...mostly me) hasn't the discipline to continue working with concepts we don't enjoy. I doubt forced effort would yield sustainable, desirable results anyway.

   Engaging in any activity that isn't genuine or consistent with one's beliefs usually results in the effort becoming sporadic, then abandoned, with staff and patients growing confused as to one's true conviction. (Engaging in such unauthentic and ineffective efforts results from a failure to clarify values.) I wish this were an audio book, if there is such a thing. Then I could just SCREAM **clarify your values**, about every 10 minutes.

4. **Not Perceived as Advertising**--This might just be personal bias-I'm over 50 and opinionated--but that which is obviously an ad reeks of self-service. I find such distinct self-promotional efforts-no matter how cleverly disguised--embarrassing to observe, and doubt they are effective. I believe an office positioned in such a manner is seen as greedy, desperate, or both.

   This general description in hand, let's consider specific marketing plans my office employs. I believe this examination will clarify any of the above general points upon which one might be temporarily uncertain.

Chapter 7

Defining a Practice's Unique Selling Position

The first and most essential step in the development of one's marketing plan (I'm assuming value clarification has been accomplished, and beliefs vividly shared with one's team, or you're wasting your time here!) is defining what is UNIQUE about one's office. This description is referred to as the office's **Unique Selling Position** (henceforth USP).

Please take no shortcuts during this essential operation, as the fate of every marketing venture hinges on the successful implementation of this process. I'd suggest devoting at least an entire two-hour staff meeting to the topic. Our office invested months of team effort in this vital venture. Allow me to review how our USP came to be, and thus offer techniques that might prove helpful in the quest to create a USP for your practice.

Begin by requesting each staff member to prepare a written list of every positive feature they can think of that is associated with your office. Have these lists placed on your private office's desk at least a day before your next staff meeting. Assign one staff person to collect and compile these ideas, eliminating duplication, to form one master list. Use a large pad of paper (big enough for the entire staff to read during the team meeting) on which to record these coalesced advantages, before the meeting begins.

During the staff meeting, discuss and enlarge on each office benefit (piggybacking on others' ideas). Have one staff member combine similar ideas, and eliminate those considered inaccurate or not unique (using local anesthetic is not worthy of mention--even in Iowa!--but being able to consistently give painless injections and dependably providing profound numbness certainly is), to arrive at a definitive list of the positive features of your office.

THE BENEFITS BEQUEATHED FROM THESE FEATURES ARE WHAT ONE MARKETS.

Our USP follows. It was helpful to our thought process to divide our office features into categories of:

Cost--Comfort--Convenience--Value.

Our USP should not be your USP, as our procedures and values will differ from yours. Study our efforts with an eye on identifying the USP of your office. PLEASE NOTICE how every marketing effort we'll examine in the remainder of this segment flows directly from the results of this essential office value clarification process.

Unique Selling Position

COST

1. Providing written estimates for each patient, before any definitive treatment, eliminates any unpleasant financial uncertainty and surprises.
2. Cash and senior citizen discounts are available.
3. Financing is available.
4. We firmly understand that dental health is cheap, while dental disease is expensive, and that
5. Quality dental care is a better value than inexpensive care, over time.

COMFORT

1. Pleasant, friendly, gentle, people-oriented staff who treat each patient like family.
2. FREE nitrous oxide (laughing gas) and gel to numb the gums are provided in an office famous for gentle, comfortable, predictable, and profound anesthetic.
3. Complimentary health and refreshment bar, with free exotic juice blends, soft drinks, tea, coffee, fruit and muffins, is available to patients.
4. Virtual reality glasses connected to cable TV allow dental care appointments to pass quickly and pleasantly, as one watches a favorite program or VCR tape.
5. Proper use of nitrous oxide means no shots are required to treat baby teeth.
6. Free SEGA games, toys, stickers, coloring books, coupons for French fries, sandwiches and milkshakes, and stuffed animal giveaways every month result in kids being delighted to visit

our office! (And having kids enjoy dental care profoundly reduces their parents' concerns.)

(Local fast food outlets are happy to give us an unlimited supply of food coupons, as they appreciate the effortless marketing these inexpensive items, distributed by our office, provide for their businesses. All we have to do is ask for more of these coupons, whenever we need them. I prefer milkshakes over solid foods, as I use amalgam, and one need not worry about the fracturing of new restorations.)

7. Enjoy using our warm, moist, lemon-scented towels to cleanse and refresh yourself after treatment.
8. Heated and herbal-scented orthopedic neck pillows feel great and enhance patients' comfort.

CONVENIENCE

1. Multiple dentists allow our office to be open longer hours, and some Saturdays, so convenient times are available, no matter how busy one's schedule, and every emergency patient will be seen the day he or she needs our help.
2. Insurance is submitted for patients at no charge.
3. We have an 800 number and five phone lines, so patients don't pay for calls, and don't get busy signals when they need us.
4. We provide every type of dental care, including all types of fillings, crowns, dentures, partials, oral surgery, root canals, gum treatment, orthodontics, TMJ and advanced cosmetic dentistry--so patients aren't forced to receive care in an unfamiliar specialist's office, usually many miles from home.

VALUE

1. Dr. Wilde gives a written warranty to every patient, supporting all major work. This demonstrates our commitment to quality, and removes the risk of dental care for the patient. If you're not happy, we redo the work, or refund your investment.
2. Our office is in total compliance with, or exceeds, all OSHA standards of sterilization and safety.
3. We use only the finest materials and best clinical techniques.
4. Staff dentists offer a combined 40-plus years of dental experience.
5. Dr. Wilde is an internationally known dental authority, who has had four dental books and over 100 magazine articles published. He speaks on dental topics, and is also a former University of Iowa College of Dentistry faculty member.
6. Our office is concerned about the satisfaction and well-being of every patient, treating them as kindly we would our families.

Can you envision how the benefits forthcoming from the varied facets of our USP become the basis for all office promotions? Can you detect reflected bits of our clarified practice values within these features? The creation of our USP led to a totally new concept pertaining to our Yellow Pages ad. We retained the office logo and phone number, but decided to risk life without such catchy, motivational marketing phrases as "new patients welcome"!

As you study this copy, notice how our USP is employed to highlight the **BENEFITS** one receives from seeking care in our office. At least in our geographic area, no other office Yellow Pages ad is composed as a personal letter, detailing the advantages our office provides every patient we treat.

YELLOW PAGES

"Get a Taste of Truly Gentle Dentistry"

Please come visit our **bright, cheery, modern office** where up-to-date technology is combined with the **personal touch** of caring dentists and staff. Discover modern dentistry can be uplifting, lighthearted, even fun, for adults and children.

Relax in our family-atmosphere reception area. Enjoy **complimentary snacks and beverages** from our health and refreshment bar, while your kids experience our special children's area, complete with giant Sega machine. (But don't expect to wait long--we are an **on-time office**.)

Soothing **laughing gas** means more comfort for you, **no shots for your kids**, and it's provided **FREE**. Watch cable television through our **virtual reality glasses**--something you must experience to believe--as time flies by while you receive care.

Three dentists mean **Prompt Emergency Care, and Evening and Saturday appointments**. You'll never be abandoned in time of need because no dentist is available that day--let alone for two weeks!

We feature painless, one-appointment root canals, plus the most modern in cosmetic care including bonding, veneers and easy, comfortable, affordable tooth lightening. **Today everyone may have the beautiful smile of his or her dreams!** Our infection control exceeds all requirements.

Every effort is made to **Achieve the Care You Need, Within the Framework of Your Budget**. We complete insurance forms for you, feature senior and cash discounts, have financing available and offer payment plans.

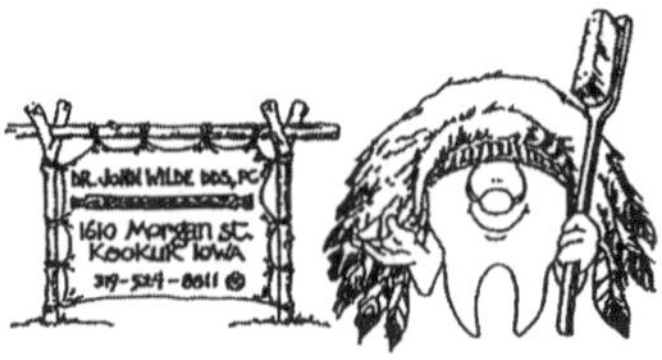

Please call **319-524-8811** or **Dial Toll Free** 1-800-742-WILD to make appointments for yourself and those you love today.

MasterCard Visa

Dr. John A. Wilde and Staff

1610 MORGAN STREET • KEOKUK, IA

It's critically important to **highlight** key features of this ad. Many people are impatient, or struggle to read. One should be able to reach an accurate and impressive idea of our office, merely by sweeping his or her eyes over accented material. (Take a second and scan our ad highlights, to see what I mean.)

When we first ran this ad, I feared it worked too well! We always ask new patients who referred them, and instead of the customary existing patients' names, we more and more frequently heard a response of "the Yellow Pages."

I much prefer a personal referral, as it is usually accompanied by a strong endorsement. It is ideal to have patients first visit one's office already enthusiastic because of a strong positive recommendation from a family member or friend. Also, by considering the patient who referred this new client to us, we gain some helpful insight into the new patient's values.

As I interviewed these new patients, a pattern emerged. As is typical in our rural area, these folks had asked friends and neighbors which dentist to see. Often they heard several names. (Keokuk is truly blessed with outstanding dentists!) No matter what practice sounds best, they needed to consult the Yellow Pages to get a phone number, and often our ad was the final bit of information that led to the call to our office.

(MANY people comment that they love the stupid little cartoon Indian logo! This was designed by an artist in Colorado I never even spoke to, the first time our office had mugs customized. I have no idea what this insipid figure is supposed to represent--it's NOT ME!--but my staff repeatedly assures me that patients seem to relate to it somehow.)

The Warsaw Letters

Inspired by the results of our Yellow Pages, I decided to employ our USP in a really unique manner for our office. We had never sent any type of direct mail messages, but I felt our USP created a solid basis upon which to build, and an unusual opportunity existed.

The town of Warsaw, Illinois--population approximately 2,000, with a much larger drawing area, located five miles south of Keokuk--had been without a dentist for over a year. We decided the timing was ideal to target some of Warsaw's residents for a direct mail marketing campaign.

I considered opening a Warsaw satellite office (having a second office location is the one mistake I've yet to make in dentistry, remember?), and with a third dentist just coming aboard, we had the doctor time available for such an undertaking.

Direct mail--bring them to us--might not be as effective as opening an office in Warsaw, but it's one hell of a lot cheaper, and certainly less fraught with financial peril. (And losing money, of any amount, makes me grumpy!)

The ADA sells lists of dentists' names, addresses and phone numbers to multiple companies who are delighted to peddle versions of this compilation to anyone. Call the ADA (1-800-621-8099) and they will provide the names and numbers of these list-selling companies. (Be sure to contact several companies and get precise, written bids. To my surprise, the cost of purchasing identical ADA-provided lists of dentists varied by up to 100 percent!)

I'd used these companies to provide lists of dentists to whom I marketed my books. These same businesses, with the assistance of modern computers, sell lists of people's names and addresses conforming to any and every possible description and parameter. For our direct mail project, we asked for the names and addresses of all in the Warsaw area zip codes with annual incomes in excess of $30,000. This request resulted in a list of 568 households.

We inhabit a world where information is power. These lists can be created to meet your precise specifications. I could have requested only left-handed redheads currently involved in their third marriage, who own tropical fish--but I assume the list would have been shorter!

Had I the opportunity to select my target population over again, I would include everyone over age 55. I think we missed a lot of senior citizens, due to the annual income limitation, and I consider these seasoned folks to be wonderful patients. (Many seniors might fall below our annual income goal, yet have access to substantial financial resources, and they are the primary population for the removable prosthodontics I enjoy.)

No office can serve everyone well. The value clarification process helps your team identify the type of folks with whom you feel most comfortable, and thus are best able to offer dental care. The description of one's list criteria should be carefully and accurately defined, to reflect office values and ideally preferred type of patient--young families, seniors, wealthy, middle class, etc.--upon which one's office focuses. (As you can see, I dropped the ball badly for my practice by overlooking seniors.)

We wanted to send a carefully crafted series of four letters, so we ordered four sets of pre-stick labels. The total cost of labels was $493 plus shipping. (One can also order a computer disc and print labels yourself, which is cheaper, provides better control, and the disc serves as a permanent record. I was unaware of this option at the time I placed my order--or maybe too technophobic to try this, I can't remember for sure--but I'd order a disc if doing multiple mailings today.)

We mailed roughly 2,272 letters. (Four times 568 = 2,272.) I estimate our out-of-pocket expense (printing, stationery and postage) to be about $.50 per letter, so our total cash outlay was $493 for the list and $1,136 printing and mailing, for a sum of $1,629. Of course, staff time to prepare the mailing, and the cost of the free examination and bitewing x-rays offered, must also be considered.

During the three months of mailings (we posted the series of four letters at three-week intervals), and the month following, we scheduled 16 new patients who received $17,558 worth of care--almost 11 times our out-of-pocket cost. With our 48 percent overhead, our net was approximately $8,700...a **534 percent return on investment in about six months' time!** ($8,700 / $1,629 = 534 percent) And I thought the stock market was doing well!

As I've mentioned, I'd prefer to be able to document an immediate profit from marketing. But this initial return represents but the tip of the iceberg. In the months and years to come, these patients will need additional care, and I hope these satisfied families will also refer their friends and neighbors. I also anticipate that when others, who received the letters but didn't act immediately, require future dental care, they will remember our messages and call for appointments. (A dentist named Wilde isn't too hard to recollect!) Since the initial restorative care was measured, we have completed two full ortho cases on these patients, for about $6,000 in additional production.

The focus of the following letters is on **benefits** to the patient (drawn from our USP) and dental health **education**. Please note we carefully and repeatedly advised patients who were pleased with their existing dentist to stay in their happy dental homes. To the best of my knowledge, none of the patients we saw currently had a dentist.

Each letter contained educational handouts (a brief description of each follows the letter with which it was sent) and a full page of **patient testimonials**. Of course, we used different testimonials with each letter.

The letters took a long time to craft. Please feel free to copy or modify them as you see fit, if such an undertaking seems appropriate and worthwhile to you.

PLEASE DON'T SKIMP ON YOUR EFFORTS TO OBTAIN TESTIMONIALS! I had a staff member (the head of our PR efforts) request patients--ones we valued and enjoyed--to write these powerful messages. (A dentist with less fear of rejection could ask for himself or herself.)

We chose our testimonial targets with care, selecting patients with whom we related well. Everyone we asked agreed to write something, although some efforts were better suited to our purpose than others. We sent an office mug filled with sugarless candy and a sincere note of thanks to each patient kind enough to pen a testimonial, whether we used it or not. If nothing else, these generous messages warmed my heart...even if we had to ask for them. (My generic advice to dentists: enjoy compliments any way you can get them. There's little risk of us overdosing on them!)

First Warsaw Letter

"A VALUE OF UP TO $500 FOR YOUR ENTIRE FAMILY-FREE!"

Dear Neighbor,

I'd like to take a moment in this too-busy world to introduce our office, and talk to you friend to friend. And like any good neighbor, I'd like to offer you some sound advice about achieving excellent oral health. It's a topic I've studied for over 30 years. (If you're confused by my youthful good looks, I confess I entered dental school when I was 8 years old.)

This advice concerns the number-one reason people's "teeth" become plastic things soaking in a cup beside the bed at night. That villain is periodontal, or gum disease. **Almost certainly you or someone you love has active gum disease right now!**

The early signs are seldom painful, and consist mainly of bleeding gums (ALWAYS a sign of an existing active bacterial infection), bad breath (hard on both business and personal life), and finally loose and sore teeth with painful, pus-filled gum abscesses that quickly lead to tooth loss.

For those suffering from gum disease, time is critical, as the infection is destroying your jawbone. Often early, simple treatment can prevent or cure gum disease, but the problem must be caught in time.

As if you didn't have enough to worry about, recent medical studies have linked periodontal and heart disease. Need further motivation? The eminent physician, **Dr. Charles Mayo, stated that a healthy mouth can add 10 to 15 years to a person's life.** (The bad news is it's always added at the end. I'd prefer to have the extra years at about age 25!!)

How about some good news to follow all that dentist babble? **Today Almost Everyone Can Keep Their Natural Teeth in Health and Comfort for a Lifetime!** But, you need a dentist's help.

If you have a dentist, go see him or her. If you don't have a happy dental home, I'd like to offer our services to you. As a good neighbor, I'm going to make this proposal in a manner that eliminates all your risk by offering your family a **FREE DENTAL HEALTH EXAM**. And I don't mean just a quick look around your mouth, but bitewing x-rays, gum check, blood pressure, oral cancer exam (a quick, easy, painless procedure that could save your life!), and cosmetic evaluation (we can do amazing things for your smile today). This can represent an **enormous savings of up to $500 per family**.

This is a No Risk, No Cost, No Obligation way to meet the friendly dental family at John A. Wilde, D.D.S., P.C. Please call TOLL FREE 1-800-742-WILD and let us welcome you to our happy dental family of 4,723 patients (and growing!)

Sincerely,

Staff of John A. Wilde, D.D.S., P.C.

P.S. We are a busy dental office, so there is a limit to how many "let's get acquainted," free exams we can perform. Please call immediately to avoid being placed on a waiting list!

Included with this mailing was a page of patient testimonials, a one-page article reprinted from *Consumer Reports* discussing periodontal disease and possible treatments, and a dental magazine article examining the possible link between periodontal and heart disease. The figure for our patient population--4,723--was the number our computer registered as patients of record the day the letter was written.

Of course, as patients called to schedule appointments, their address stickers were removed from our master list, so no further mailings were sent them.

Second Warsaw Letter
"THE SECRETS OF A BEAUTIFUL SMILE"

Dear Neighbor,

Hi. It's John Wilde again--the dentist who wrote a few weeks ago about periodontal disease and your dental health. We've heard from plenty of your neighbors--we've been burning some "midnight oil" (working after 5 p.m. for a dentist) performing their "get acquainted" exams. It's been great fun, but we missed you, and we're concerned. The best reason for not calling is you already have a dentist you love, and that's great! We wouldn't want to alter a positive dentist-patient relationship for anything in the world. But if some other reason has kept you from making an appointment, please listen to me once again.

The enclosed postcard is pretty dramatic. Look in the bathroom mirror, and see which of these two images your mouth most closely resembles. Our office did a "scientific study" and discovered most folks don't prefer black teeth.

Let me get straight to the point: **Modern dentistry allows virtually everyone to have the smile they've always dreamed of! Bonding** can make teeth look whiter, straighter, repair chips or close spaces and **is done without shots or cutting of teeth. Porcelain veneers straighten teeth without braces** and are three times as strong as natural teeth. We offer **comfortable, simple, affordable tooth lightening** to return your teeth to the color they were when you were sixteen. (Sorry, nothing I can do for the rest of your body. Sooner or later, gravity seems to win!)

Cosmetic dentistry can improve your career, increase your

self-confidence and self-esteem, making you a happier, easier-to-meet person. Modern materials give us the opportunity to dramatically improve patients' lives. Even dentists have to get excited about that!

Excellent modern dental care isn't cheap, but our office will do everything possible to allow you to **receive the care you desire within the limits of your budget**. We offer cash and senior discounts and accept credit cards. **Written estimates are given before any major treatment is performed**, and financing is available.

How you look, how you smile, affects every part of your life. There is no need to tolerate a smile that is less than ideal. Call **toll-free for a FREE EXAMINATION (at an enormous savings of up to $500 per family) at 1-800-742-WILD.**

Sincerely,

Staff of John A. Wilde, D.D.S., P.C.

P.S. We are so excited about seeing you that we are offering a **FREE DENTAL HEALTH KIT** to every patient. The kit includes an excellent toothbrush, toothpaste, floss and several other goodies. (We enjoy spoiling our guests!)

Along with a new page of testimonials, we included a postcard from High Impact Images showing a before and after photo of a quadrant, first with amalgam, then composite restorations. Phone 719-488-0808 to receive a copy of High Impact Images' brochure displaying their incredible dental photography.

Third Warsaw Letter
"DON'T FOOLISHLY RISK THE LIVES OF YOU AND YOUR LOVED ONES!"

Dear Neighbor,

John Wilde again. We've been swamped by calls from your friends and neighbors responding to our $500-per-family free exam offer. But, tired as we are, I'm still concerned we haven't heard from you, as my goal is for everyone in the area to enjoy excellent oral health in a happy dental home. As the enclosed article from Melinda Beeler's paper, *The Connection*, points out, **Not Having a Dental Examination Can KILL YOU!**

Most of us know oral cancer patients or victims. Thirty thousand Americans a year contract this disease, and 8,000 of them die. **That's one American death per hour from oral cancer!** Everyone should have an annual oral cancer exam, but those who use tobacco and/or alcohol are **High-Risk Candidates**. If these letters do nothing else, at least be sure you and yours are checked for this deadly killer. An oral cancer examination is quick, easy, painless and could save your life.

I'm sorry if talk of cancer frightens you. It's a word all of us dread. For too many the word "dentistry" is also alarming, but **I'm here to tell you fearing dental care no longer makes sense!** I'll admit having dental work performed is less fun than eating ice cream, **BUT DENTISTRY DOESN'T HURT ANY MORE.**

Using gels to numb the gums before shots, combined with free laughing gas, has allowed our office to become famous for **gentle, comfortable, predictable and profound anesthesia.** (That's the title of an article I had published in one of America's most-read dental journals.) With laughing gas, **your kids don't need shots to fill baby teeth**, and they won't feel a thing, except a pleasant, floaty feeling.

Cable TV hooked to Virtual Reality glasses is something you have to experience to believe! It really helps distract kids and grownups alike during dental care, making time seem to fly by, as well as significantly diminishing sounds of the drill.

FREE GIANT SEGA, special play area, stickers, toys, activity books, free milkshake, French-fry and sandwich coupons make our office a place kids bring their friends along to experience. We have an "adult toy box" filled with pleasant surprises too (to reward a grownup, in case one is ever well-behaved). Everyone is invited to help themselves to our **free health and refreshment bar** featuring coffee, tea, soft drinks, juice, fruit and muffins--even home-made bread, baked fresh right in our office every day! (We love the smell!)

The real key to comfortable dental care is our staff. Relax in our office and find the care you need--no more, no less--among warm, friendly, gentle people who treat every patient as members of their family. We can't offer these $500 free exams much longer. We hope you'll call toll-free 1-800-742-WILD to make an appointment.

Sincerely,

The Staff of John A. Wilde, D.D.S., P.C.

P.S. If you're just not certain about our generous offer and wish to stop by, say hello, tour our office and get to know us, we'd be happy to give you one of our free dental health kits, just for dropping by.

Different testimonials and a copy of an article I wrote about oral cancer, previously published in the Warsaw local newspaper, were included with this mailing. We did have one nice lady "drop in" our office, just to check us out. Yes, she became a very nice patient.

Fourth Warsaw Letter
"FINAL OFFER"

Dear Neighbor,

Our supply of **free dental health kits** and time available to offer our **$500 free dental examinations** are almost exhausted. It's been fun meeting your friends and neighbors, but the response has been so tremendous, **I doubt we'll ever be able to make an offer like this again!** Still, our goal is for everyone in this area to find a happy dental home, and I wanted to make one last effort to improve the oral health of you and yours.

Consider what you've learned about **oral cancer, gum disease, the modern wonder of modern cosmetic dental care and the scientific advances that have made treatment so comfortable.** We are holding our offer open for **ONE MORE WEEK**. You still have a chance to SAVE **pain**, SAVE **expense**, SAVE **health**, SAVE **appearance** and SAVE **self-esteem**. But you must call 1-800-742-WILD today to make your no-cost, no-obligation, free examination appointment. We hope to hear from you soon, and wish you the very best. This is truly a once-in-a-lifetime opportunity!

Sincerely,

The Staff of John A. Wilde, D.D.S., P.C.

P.S. A warranty, such as the sample enclosed, is given to every patient I treat. I know of no other dental office that demonstrates such absolute faith in the quality of their care.

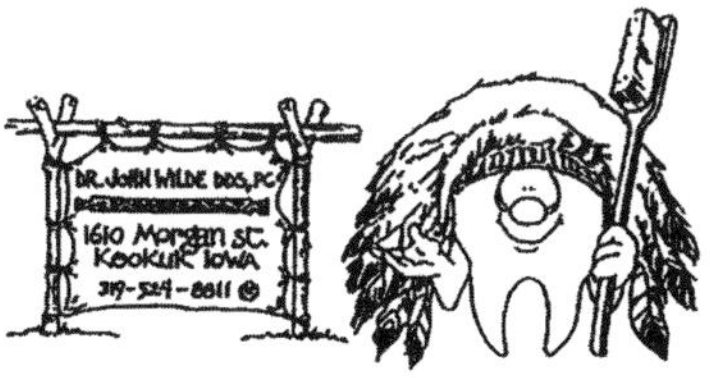

LIMITED WARRANTY

CROWN OR BRIDGE

People always ask us how long should this last. In our office we strive for perfection and satisfaction. Which is why we are happy to provide you this warranty, something no other office is offering. Let us remember in today's technology almost everything we have learned is on the preventive side. Instead of going to the dentist every few years for "Drill, Bill and Fill," let's try preventive dentistry. If you spend 4 minutes in the morning and 4 minutes in the evening brushing, flossing and doing any other special treatments your dentist and hygienist have recommended and let your dentist or hygienist professionally clean your teeth, check for decay, apply a fluoride treatment, or apply sealants, you can prevent most all disease. This is why all of your warranties must be null and void if we don't see you for your regular 6-month check-ups. With 6-month check-ups your teeth and gums are winners!

1. FOR A PERIOD OF 3 YEARS FROM THE DATE OF SERVICE, WE WILL REFUND THE COST OF A CROWN OR BRIDGE DUE TO BREAKAGE, MISFIT, OR DECAY AT NO COST TO THE PATIENT.*

2.THIS WARRANTY IS NULL AND VOID IF THE PATIENT DOES NOT MAINTAIN HIS/HER 6-MONTH CONTINUING CARE CLEANING APPOINTMENTS.

* GOLD AND PORCELAIN CROWNS ARE THE SAME FOR PRACTICALLY ALL CASES EXCEPT THAT PORCELAIN CAN CHIP. APPROXIMATELY 1 OUT OF EVERY 100 PORCELAIN CROWNS WILL CHIP AND NEED REPLACING. THIS WILL NEVER HAPPEN WITH GOLD CROWNS. IF YOUR PORCELAIN CROWN CHIPS IN THE FIRST 3 YEARS WE WILL REPLACE IT FOR FREE. HOWEVER, IF IT CHIPS AFTER THE 3-YEAR PERIOD IT WOULD COST YOU THE REGULAR FEE FOR A NEW CROWN. THIS SHOULD BE TAKEN IN CONSIDERATION WHEN CHOOSING BETWEEN A PORCELAIN AND A GOLD CROWN.

I'd like to confess this warranty was stolen verbatim from the excellent work of my friend, Dr. Howard Farran, boy-wonder, dental genius, writer, speaker, now even a personal fitness expert...a man for all seasons!! (Although, come to think of it, Howard lives in Arizona, where they basically have but one season! I could possibly understand misplacing one season, but losing three smacks of pure carelessness! At least Howard is a man for one season.)

We have different warranties for every type of major dental procedure we perform. The warranty is handed to the patient as the treatment plan is being discussed--not after treatment is complete--as I believe this concrete expression of our confidence and character significantly increases case acceptance.

No one can **guarantee results** (a phrase dentists should completely avoid). But I stand behind my treatment, and have from my first days in practice--written warranty or no--and will refund or re-treat any care with which a patient is unhappy. If you share a similar commitment to accept nothing short of the best you can provide, why not take advantage of your professionalism and fairness by offering a warranty for your work?

Here is one example of the page of testimonial(s) we sent with each of the four letters. Now, my mother raised no fools. This letter is clearly the pick of the litter. (That's Iowa-speak for best.) I was moved to tears when I first read this. It was written by a delightful lady after we crowned her remaining six lower anterior teeth, then fabricated a precision lower partial and upper denture.

How I envy this wonderful lady her writing ability! I'd like to send this letter with every mailing--I'd like to have it blown up and put on a billboard downtown--but we used a fresh testimonial page with each of the four letters. (Most testimonials were much shorter than the following masterpiece, so three or four were included--whatever fit comfortably on a single page.)

"Very few face the prospect of visiting their dentist joyfully, especially when the appointment was created to take care of dental problems.

My experience, however, with the office of my dentist, Dr. John Wilde, has changed all of that.

Presented with my mouthful of dental challenges, Dr. Wilde and his staff rose to the occasion. During each visit, I was made to feel like I was visiting with an old friend, while within my mouth, five root canals were performed, an entire set of bottom caps were created and positioned into place, as well as additional preventative and recreative procedures were followed. Even when faced with extraction of a tooth, a procedure generally referred to a specialist, Dr. Wilde, and his associate, Dr. Long, painlessly removed the tooth.

As an older woman, on my own, I appreciate those who sincerely are looking out for my best interest. As my dentist, Dr. Wilde only prescribes treatments that are necessary. If there are other, more costly procedures that could provide some benefit, I am given the option to choose, without any pressure. If I am not completely certain, there is always a chance to think and consider. My comfort and ease remain top priority, not only with my dentist, but also with every member of his staff.

The greatest gift I have been given, however, is not Dr. Wilde's excellent dental care: it is the tremendous human compassion that is extended in every encounter. In our high gloss, high pressure world, it is easy for people to be herded rather than helped, processed rather than sensitively touched. By his gracious and humble manner, my life has been enriched. Yes, I have greater dental health than I have had for years, but more importantly, I have been encouraged to expect the best out of life.

Dentist visits no longer are faced with fear, but with the knowledge that I will leave the office benefited, orally and emotionally. For that experience, I am sincerely grateful."

(No! This lovely patient was not my mother!)

As mentioned, these letters were a one-time event in my career. The voice--the "high intensity sales pitch tone"--came from the marketing expert whose course I took, and whose advice I followed. I believe long-term practice prosperity depends on providing consistently outstanding care, offered in a comfortable environment, by behaviorally skilled professionals. This combination of behaviors leads to relationships that are the foundation upon which all successful businesses depend.

If one is beginning a practice, needs additional growth, or is undergoing a rapid change--such as implementing expanded hygiene, or adding an associate--such marketing efforts can provide a quick boost in new patient numbers. But an office must routinely provide every benefit it describes, or patients won't return. I have no problem with marketing--dental or otherwise--but performance, not conversation, is the key to long-term dental success. As we note in the Heartland, there's a lot of difference between being a bull and a steer. (Don't fret about this. You'll get it or you won't, but I'm not explaining.)

Chapter 8

Office Promotions, Chart Audit and PR Calendar

As we continue to examine ideas to enhance patient flow to one's practice, I'm going to use our No-Cavity Club as an illustration of the type of marketing activity we enjoy, and believe to be valuable. As the PR calendar at the end of this chapter will attest, the No-Cavity Club is one of many such promotional activities we routinely offer, including Senior Month, Children's Dental Health Month, coloring contests and many more. I choose to describe the No-Cavity Club in detail, as it may be our most effective practice enhancement vehicle (thanks to a somewhat unique twist we add to this well-discussed concept), and accurately represents the general principles underlying the great majority of our marketing efforts.

THE NO-CAVITY CLUB

This undertaking fits our office's generic description of an ideal marketing venture almost perfectly:

a) It's **simple** to do.

b) It's a lot of **fun** for staff, parents and especially our young patients.

c) The **cost is minimal**--four quality stuffed animals a year. (My wife purchases them at someplace like Wal-Mart.)

d) The **impact** on our patients, practice and community is **significant**.

e) **It doesn't SEEM TO BE ADVERTISING**.

We have a HUGE STUFFED ANIMAL (don't save a few bucks here, go for maximum impact with the largest, most outrageous specimen you can buy!) sitting in our reception room with a sign around its neck stating, "**KIDS,** you can win me in the No-Cavity Club drawing!" Members of our club include:

1. All children who have perfect check-ups.
2. **Kids for whom we recommend treatment, after they have ALL their care completed.**

Can you imagine kids pestering parents to get their dental work done, so they can be included in the drawing? As we've mentioned, and will examine more fully later, we use only nitrous oxide--no shots-to restore primary teeth, so kids feel floaty and happy, ENJOYING their dental experience.

When kids "qualify as club members," they, their parents or one of our staff fill out a card stating the child's name and phone number, then drop it into our special No-Cavity Club drawing box (a shoebox covered with shiny wrapping paper, with a rectangular hole cut in the top).

Every three months we have a "drawing," to determine the stuffed critter's new owner. (This is often rigged, as staff will have selected a child in advance, who, for whatever reason, they feel most deserves to have the toy animal. I've never won an argument with any woman, so I protest such injustice but mildly, then, like Pilate, wash my hands of responsibility for this tainted contest!)

To this point, we've had some fun and added energy and excitement to a mundane office. **The next segment of our project adds an additional step to this venerable idea, and leverages its impact significantly.**

The name of each child entered in our contest is typed, and a short note added to this list, congratulating all "No-Cavity Club winners" for their perfect mouths, and stressing the importance of good oral health in children. The local paper sends a reporter, who accepts our prepared list of names and our message, takes a picture of our winner, the stuffed animal (usually at least the size of the kid) and one or two smiling staff members. (We select staff who don't resemble the stuffed animal too closely, to avoid confusion. I haven't been in a picture yet! I think the problem concerns the shape of my ears.)

How do you get such items published in the paper without paying for an advertisement? By working at it. Understanding this fact helps: Newspapers are black holes that must be filled each day by harried reporters and editors. Local news, like our contest, is free and of more interest to local residents than a generic news story purchased from a wire service. It seems everyone enjoys reading about people they know. Also, photographs--especially ones of smiling kids with huge stuffed animals--grab reader attention, while filling a lot of blank newspaper space.

Take time to develop a relationship with a local reporter. You or your staff may already know someone, or even have a newspaper staff member as a patient. You, or your PR director, might invest in lunch with the reporter, exploring how this news professional would prefer to work with your office. Go out of your way to accommodate his or her schedule, and do all you can--as preparing lists, typing copy, organizing people for the picture--to make his or her job simple.

These newsprint folks, at least in our area, are way overworked, and way underpaid.

This concept might not work for the *New York Times*, but smaller community papers, shoppers, even school papers are possible sources for such a venture, and exist almost everywhere. We have an article, usually including a photograph, in our local paper concerning an office event almost every month. (When I retired, my photo and an article about my career comprised the top half of the local paper's front page! Most dentists would have to be busted for a pretty juicy offense to get such press! It can be fun to have friends in the news industry....Or perhaps getting rid of me was considered a cause for community celebration?)

The No-Cavity Club photo, along with our note of congratulations, and all the kids' names, is published in the Big Wednesday Business Section of our local paper. Even children who don't win the animal get the thrill of seeing their name in the paper. How many of these articles do you think are clipped and hung on the refrigerator?

The contest is kept going constantly, and along with our world-class toy chest, GIANT SEGA MACHINE in the reception area, stickers, craft books, free milkshake, sandwiches and French fry coupons, and our genuine enjoyment of these special little patients, makes our office a very popular place for kids to visit, **bringing along their friends and parents**. (We often have kids drop in to play in our office while one of their parents is having a medical appointment in a near-by office. We think it's cool!)

Our office has had articles featuring our virtual reality glasses, intra-oral camera system, new associate dentists or team members joining the office (certainly including hygienist and hygiene assistant), continuing education courses taken, books I've had published, and many more appear in our local daily paper. I also wrote an oral health column for an area weekly paper for about two years (from which the oral cancer article included with the Warsaw letters came). People read these smaller papers carefully to discover information (and gossip) about their community, friends and neighbors.

The key to developing such wonderful, free and effective advertising is developing a warm relationship with one member of the local paper's staff. This person must come to know and like your office, and to appreciate all the help you provide them in doing their job. The right relationship is good for the community, the paper, the reporter (who needs stuff to report)...and one's practice.

Patient Retainment

I must include the obligatory spiel--the one I've heard too many lectures opine--to the effect that when an office satisfies the patients' every wish and whim, it is rewarded by gobs of money being thrown its way, new patients are referred in herds, and staff are downright inconvenienced by the perpetual adulation--if not outright worship--of the masses.

No patient ever leaves such an office of behavioral wonder, even after moving off the continent, let alone to save a few bucks on some third-party insurance plan! (Want to have the most patients of any office in your area and be loved by all? WORK FOR FREE!)

This requisite praise to patient service rendered, take a cleansing breath, and let's return to reality. Every dental office--yes, even those whose dentists lecture--loses patients. Even the most behaviorally aware can't control the actions of others, only guide them. For reasons of illness, lost jobs, personal tragedy, simple forgetfulness, or becoming angry at our practice or a specific staff member--patients will "fall through the cracks" of the most efficient office. Due to these facts, **CHART AUDIT**--the effort to restore failed relationships between patients and one's practice--is a perpetual task, and a valuable tool, that helps achieve our office objectives.

Chart Audit

One must ask staff to face rejection when performing chart audit. This is a risk only a very few brave people feel comfortable taking. Calling out-of-touch patients to encourage them to schedule an appointment means deliberately placing oneself in a position to be told "no." This negative response can be perceived, not just as a refusal of offered dental care, but as a denial of the very individual posing the oft-tremulous query.

Because of this fear of rejection, chart audit is always among the last jobs undertaken by hard-working dental team members. (Sort of the toilet scrubbing of dentistry...necessary, but unpleasant.) Yet, keeping in touch with patients of record, especially in situations such as when one is trying to rapidly expand a hygiene department, is an essential portion of realizing optimal practice success. So let's consider a **system** that can assure the office leader this important, but difficult task is continuously and skillfully performed.

There exist three essential ingredients for successful chart audit--one must have a leader, a team, and a clearly defined system. Let's consider the various facets of this perpetual process, as implemented in our office.

1. **Leader**--The dentist provides the over-arching office vision, and develops appropriate systems, but a single staff person must coordinate and monitor all chart audit efforts. This person is a champion--a prized jewel within the office--and should be acknowledged and rewarded as such. (Given public praise and private money.) This leader might emerge from the ranks of hygiene, the front office, be your PR coordinator,

even a dentist. He or she must be someone who understands human behavior, possesses organizational ability, has excellent communication skills and works effectively with others. (In all candor, the above somewhat daunting description eliminates 99.9 percent of dentists from consideration for the task.)

2. **Team**--We'll detail possible team members when we consider the system, during Step 4 of our examination.
3. **Effective Dialogue**--Before placing any calls, a chart audit person must carefully review each patient's record. Dialing numbers--calling patients cold--is a painful exercise in futility, and doesn't portray one's office in the caring light most dentists would desire. Specific facts, both personal and dental, are gleaned from the patient's record before any call is made.

We routinely note personally meaningful information like special vacations, hobbies, birth of a child, pets, etc. in the permanent treatment record, as such information helps us establish a deeper bond with patients. (In pre-computer days, we noted such information on the patient's chart in green ink-a special green pen was left in every treatment area--so this data really jumped out at you. This was one of about a million outstanding ideas Dr. Earl Estep suggested.)

It is pretty impressive to our clients when, six months or a year later, staff can remember such notable details. (Personally, I'm impressed with myself when I can recall such facts as today's date, what I ate for my last meal, or my parent's phone number.) Often, recalling these personal insights is a great "ice-breaker," and helps reestablish rapport with a patient temporarily out of contact with one's office. Such attention to detail demonstrates that we regard patients as individuals, not just names with which to fill our schedule...or our wallets.

Armed with this personal and dental awareness, a typical call might begin, "Hi, Tom. This is Kathy from Dr. Wilde's office? **DR. WILDE ASKED ME TO CALL**. It's been 18 months since we checked your teeth! At that time, we noted an area of possibly developing decay on the upper right, and **DR. WILDE IS CONCERNED**. Have you been experiencing any dental problems?"

The exact phrases, "Dr. Wilde asked me to call...he's concerned" work like magic! I'm uncertain why, but suspect patients respond to the idea of a busy dentist fretting about them. Technically, I'm not aware that Kathy is calling this patient at this precise moment. Generically, I am very concerned about any patient who has slipped away from regular care, having witnessed the painful, expensive dental disasters that occur due to such neglect countless times.

I would suggest a very precise chart audit dialogue be developed by one's team, and role-played among staff until all are comfortable. Of course, each staff person should express his or her concern in a natural manner. But, while form may vary, the CONTENT of each message should be similar, irrespective of who is making the call. (There does exist one best way to say anything, and this ideal form must be identified and practiced until it feels completely comfortable.)

The clinical comment might concern bleeding gums, pocketing, or reminding the patient of the terrible toothache he or she previously suffered, and explaining we wouldn't want them to be forced to deal with excruciating pain and threatening infections like that ever again. (Reinforcing and deepening this experience is a powerful behavioral technique.) A wisdom tooth that has concerned us, a tooth we suggested be crowned, or a bridge placed might be the topic we'd discuss.

If the patient responds, "I've been meaning to call" (yeah, right!), we schedule an appointment and our task is complete. However, if there is any hint of resistance, we'll gently inquire to discover if the patient has any **unaddressed questions or concerns.** Perhaps he or she is fearful about some aspect of recommended care, feels we messed up the insurance in the past, or doesn't like the dentist's breath. (Hey, I use Scope all the time! And halitosis is better than no breath! Although I will confess to an unsightly and burgeoning nasal hair bouquet. It makes my eyes tear to yank them out! Perhaps injecting Nair? Or a flash nose-fire?)

If problems can be identified, they can be addressed and corrected. If our chart audit caller has the necessary talent and training to allow patients to trust her, and thus express their unhappiness, one has an invaluable opportunity to solve whatever is perceived to be the difficulty, and assure the patient our office will make every effort to be certain this terrible event (it was terrible to the patient) doesn't happen again. (Need I add this concern, and the proposed resolution, are entered into the patient's permanent record?)

The staff members making these calls must be positive (to deal with rejection), and possess excellent people and phone skills. But dentistry is a service business. Why would anyone hire a staff member that didn't fit this description?

If a patient advises us he is seeing another dentist, the staff person makes every effort to find a specific reason for this decision. Any concerns or comments are noted, and this information clipped to the front of the record. **The record of each patient who leaves our office, along with a copy of the most recent notes explaining why he or she left, is placed on my desk.**

I don't enjoy examining these failed relationships, but the knowledge gained from studying why a patient chose to leave our care is necessary, vital to assimilate, to allow our office to learn and improve. If a pattern of similar responses indicates a recurring problem, the system driving away patients must be examined and behavior not consistent with practice values reconfigured.

I review each individual's problem, if any, and send a form letter to every departing patient with thanks for allowing us to be of service, and assuring him or her they will be welcomed back into our happy dental family at any time. (Again, I have way too much fear of rejection to personally call each patient and discuss why they're leaving our office--although I admire the hell out of dentists who possess such strength and courage!)

The letter thanking patients for their past support, and offering to help them in any way possible in the future, is IMPORTANT! We find many patients return to our practice, often after being disappointed, or suffering pain in another office. If not for the letter, they might feel embarrassed at leaving, and worry they are no longer welcome in one's practice. Our patients begin to believe all dentists give painless shots, and generally no longer hurt patients. I wish they were right, although I'd have to lower our fees if it were true.

4. **The System**--(Always the key!) We request our entire front office team of three, plus the hygiene assistant, to each make

five chart audit calls per day. This is a target of 100 calls a week. (Four staff x five days x five calls = 100.)

We also have a monthly chart audit party where, from among the entire staff, five volunteers (we have five phone lines) spend from 5 to 7 p.m. doing nothing but making **chart audit calls**.

The office provides food: pizza, Chinese take-out--or Jo cooks. (My expanding girth is proof of my wife's culinary expertise!! You'd have to taste her Chukar (a game bird) Dijon on noodles to believe it!) We give participating staff prizes for first, second and third most patients scheduled--either cash or gifts that Jo selects. (My preference in gifts tends toward things like filleting knives, duck calls, fishing lures or similar objects I'm told are not highly esteemed by the ladies of my office. That's about all the stuff they sell where I shop.) We do everything within our power to make this a fun evening, celebrating with every scheduled patient! Of course, all staff are paid for their time, even while dining.

This chart audit party gives the hygienist an opportunity to personally help fill her schedule. In an efficient office, the hygienist should be too busy to call patients during the day. But, if the hygienist doesn't stay to support teammates during this two hours a month, how can the doctor ask staff to be concerned about filling hygiene time? To explain to a team member why she should work late to fill open hygiene time, when the hygienist has left, by stating "it's your job to stay," falls a bit short of behavioral excellence. As our hygienist's pay is based on her production, a full schedule is important to her financial well-being. Thus it shouldn't prove difficult to engage the hygienist's enthusiastic support of chart audit parties.

5. **Monitors**--AGAIN, measured behavior improves. We've had each chart audit participant record her daily calls (goal of five per day) on personal monitors, and also written the results on a team blackboard, left on display in the front office. Both systems work well, **as long as the dentist reviews and comments on each team member's chart audit performance**. I place more emphasis on calls made than on appointments scheduled--on effort over result--as I don't wish to add increased pressure to this already challenging task.

Take a deep breath and stretch. (If you think you're tired, you ought to try writing a book!) What follows is a CRITICAL POINT. While a leader can and should delegate **authority**--for example, having others make chart audit calls--he or she must **never delegate responsibility**. This is a universal law, one example of which happens to be illustrated by chart audit. Staff have been granted the authority to make calls, but the dentist has the ultimate responsibility to be sure phone contact is being made, and performed in a professional manner that represents the office in a positive light.

Tax work or personal finances are examples of two other critical areas where one may hire professional help and invest them with the authority to perform tasks, but the dentist must, at all times, keep a death grip on the reality that one must retain personal responsibility for the results. If this lesson is unclear, think it through. When you fail this test--and almost all of us have at times; certainly number me among the guilty--the resulting lessons are invariably painful and costly.

In our current example, if one forfeits responsibility and doesn't monitor, encourage, insist on precisely defined and monitored chart audit efforts being made consistently, they will gradually grind to a complete stop. **SYSTEMS not consistently monitored and reinforced DON'T EXIST!** The dentist will usually only realize this when he or she notices the hygienist is spending more time drinking coffee than treating patients.

We post the names of all who participated in the chart audit party, and the prizewinners, on the laboratory wall. This acknowledgement is another form of monitoring--of staff commitment to our purpose, in this case. I usually thank each chart audit party participant for their support during the communication exercise that begins our regular monthly staff meeting. (Staff meeting protocol--such an essential topic--is fully detailed in *Bringing Your Practice Into Focus*.)

Hygiene's personal monitors of open time (broken down into failed, cancelled and unscheduled minutes per day and per month), which we've already reviewed, afford a clear idea of when chart audit emphasis becomes more critical. If we note even a slightly growing trend in open time, we ask staff to focus more energy on chart audit, before a serious problem achieving a full hygiene schedule occurs. It's important to always be proactive as regards filling hygiene time. It's a lot easier and more efficient to schedule a patient at his convenience sometime during the next few weeks than it is to fill time open the day one is calling. (Even when offering our 10 percent short-notice discount.)

As with all PR, chart audit must be a continual effort. If one waits until open time is on the books, it will take weeks to organize this effort and even longer before one enjoys the results. Unscheduled time and the resultant lost production, once past, can never be regained.

Consider the consequences of 10 percent unfilled time on the profitability of a typical office. Assuming a 65 percent overhead, a fully booked office has a 35 percent net. At 90 percent scheduled, net drops by approximately **28.6** percent. To someone not watching closely--or not using effective monitors--a 10 percent decrease in busyness might not be readily apparent. (This decline would represent less than one hygiene opening per day in the average office. Again, I hope you've reviewed past hygiene schedules, and have an accurate grasp of your current hygiene time utilization and productivity situation.)

Substitute your overhead percentage, and get an idea of how 10 percent open time affects your bottom line. How do you feel about absorbing something like a 28.6 percent pay cut, for the same hours worked? Do you feel strongly enough to insist on a carefully monitored chart audit system that you'll set up, and for which you'll assume ultimate responsibility? Remember, a great deal of restorative care is diagnosed in hygiene, so enhanced hygiene performance benefits the entire office's bottom line.

Even if no patients are immediately scheduled, when skillfully done, chart audit provides a way for one's office to reach out to patients and express concern and demonstrate dedication to their dental health. This added commitment to patients' dental well-being enhances a practice's reputation within the community. Also, over the years, we've witnessed hundreds of patients calling shortly after refusing a chart audit request to schedule an appointment. I suspect making patients aware of their lack of care causes them to start worrying. Worse things could happen! (Like an abscess developing into a cellulitis, or a bridge being destroyed before the patient is aware of trouble.)

Chart audit is a significant portion of our marketing effort, and should be a daily task in any office that hopes to achieve maximum potential. It's much easier (and cheaper) to reactivate patients one's previously seen than to recruit new people.

Reminding patients who once trusted, but have fallen out of

relationship with, one's office, of the risks dental neglect poses, is just one more form a practice's total commitment to patients' oral health assumes.

Public Relations Calendar

Our PR leader unfailingly dedicates a portion of every Wednesday to work on PR projects. It is critical that a specific time and place be devoted to these important efforts, and that no staff or patient interruptions are tolerated during this sequestered period. If one waits until everything else is completed to begin PR...it never gets done!

What follows is a six-month sampling of our PR calendar, with brief explanations of some events added to augment their meaning. At every staff meeting, the following month's activities are discussed, and individual team members are given specific assignments to implement upcoming events. The occurrences of the previous month are reviewed, and ideas advanced to increase their impact or enhance ease of implementation in the future.

January 7 • Newspaper announcement of No-Cavity Club, place new animal for next No-Cavity Club in reception room.

14 • Valentine coloring contest begins--snowflake.

We have a lot of coloring contests, including Easter, Christmas, Spring, and anything else we can think of. One master picture is selected, copies made and handed out to all who wish to enter. (This contest's particular picture happened to be of a snowflake...not my choice!)

Kids are divided into two age groups, basically consisting of those who color within the lines, and those who venture without. All entries are placed on our office wall, and are as colorful as the brightest fall foliage. As mentioned, the winner gets a stuffed animal that has been posed near our contest announcement sign, and their picture in the paper, along with the names of all other contestants and a snappy message penned by me regarding the importance of oral health for kids.

21 • Make Welcome Wagon calls.
Update main office bulletin board.

Welcome Wagon, in the form that sent representatives door to door, no longer exists. I've received a number of ads from companies who will market, usually with a mailing, to people new to your area. We offered free exams and bite wings, and Welcome Wagon attracted lots of fine patients into our practice over the years, and I was sorry to see them discontinue their program. I have no significant experience with other systems, but DC Marketing, led by David Stone, is a company that has greatly impressed me with their excellent people, superb products and reasonable costs. I have worked with this group, and they are whom I would contact first, were I considering beginning any external marketing venture. DC Marketing may be reached by calling 800-736-3632. I believe you'll find them knowledgeable, extremely helpful and gracious to work with, in stark contrast to so many companies today.

Key to our WW success was a personal phone call from our PR coordinator, placed about two weeks after the WW visit. Our staff member greeted these newcomers, and welcomed them to our area. She offered our team's help in any way possible, and often booked the new patient examination appointment they had been "meaning to call and make." If you try a new resident service, be sure phone numbers are included (it's difficult to find numbers for people who have just moved), and personal phone calls are made. I wouldn't expect outstanding results from just a mailing.

28 • Plan February preschool visits.

Send mugs and sugarless candy to patients who refer, and patients who completed all suggested treatment.

We have a lot of preschool groups tour our office every winter. They "ride" in the dental chair, see the light, feel the air syringe, watch "Mister Thirsty" (small suction) drink a glass of water, etc. We send a new toothbrush, a gift from our ample toy-box, free food coupon and a certificate of attendance from our office, personalized with their name, home with each child. I'd guess lots of these certificates end up on refrigerators.

Such a pleasant introduction to our profession is a substantive gift to these kids. Children who have enjoyed such visits are usually comfortable, even excited about their first actual dental examination, and eager to return to a "fun place" like a dental office. I feel this effort with kids helps our office grow, at the same time we're creating a generation of happier dental patients. (Thanks mainly to nitrous oxide, I find treating kids to be generally enjoyable and profitable. Be sure you agree, before going out of your way to market to this sometimes challenging group of patients.)

February 2 • Visit Hawthorne School AM & PM--dental talk

All our team is involved in talking to groups at schools, almost always of elementary age. Most of our staff have presented school programs. I always have fun with these classes, and hope they learn a thing or two about good oral health.

4 • Children's Dental Health Month projects

implemented

(School and preschool visits coordinated.)

11 • Judge Valentine coloring contest.

18 • Preschool tours, update bulletin board.

(We have several bulletin boards that our PR head changes frequently. We feature pictures of various patients' events--weddings, anniversaries, childbirth, etc.--news topics, announcements of general interest, dental information and all the articles about our office from the newspapers on display.)

24 • Wellness clinic for George Washington School.

25 • Preschool tours of office--Welcome Wagon calls.

26 • Preschool tour at office.

March 4 • March Madness--Mad Hatters--Kids wear special hats--take pictures.

11 • Mugs sent for referrals.

We send a personal note, along with an office mug bearing our name and logo, filled with sugarless candy, to anyone nice enough to refer a new patient to our office. We prefer these be sent to a place of work, if possible, where the mug will be noticed, and we hope commented on, by many fellow workers.

The theory behind acknowledging referrals is that if one wants behavior repeated--and in this case we sure do--reward it! Nothing shows more faith in or respect for a practice than referring a friend or loved one there. Such an act of support and respect should be praised in some manner.

18 • Update patient pictures on bulletin board.

25 • Welcome Wagon calls.

31 • *No-Cavity Club for quarter ends. Type notes, place new animal in reception area.*

April--Senior Smile month--alert all staff to take senior patients' photos.

1 • *Mugs with sugar-free jelly beans mailed.*

8 • *No-Cavity Club announcement to newspaper--schedule photo.*

15 • *Mail mugs for treatment completed, referrals.*

We also mail candy-filled mugs, and cards of thanks, to all patients who complete suggested care. Flowers are nice, but are gone in a week. We purchase mugs in bulk for about $1 each. For most people, it's hard to throw away a completely functional drinking device! A plant growing in an office mug might also work, but everything would probably be thrown away when the plant died. (And I dislike our office, no matter how subliminally, being linked to death! You can't get in much trouble with mugs and sugarless candy.)

22 • *Update bulletin board, Welcome Wagon calls*

May--Graduation Recognition month

6 • *Senior Smile winner selected. Gift certificate to restaurant ordered.*

12 • *Photo of Senior Smile winner, article in paper.*

During Senior Dental Health Month, we take a photo of every "seasoned" patient seen in our office, and display their smiling faces on one of our bulletin boards. At the end of the month, we draw names and award one senior dinner for two on us. The paper takes their photo, and includes the names of all the other "winners," the seniors with excellent oral health whom we saw that month. A blurb from me, discussing how the benefits of maintaining ideal oral health are ageless, and how important good oral function is to an active senior's lifestyle, will conclude the article.

20 • Update bulletin board

27 • Welcome Wagon calls. Mugs sent.

June--Vacation Flossing--Most unique picture

We award a prize for the most unusual or impressive photo sent to us by a patient while on vacation.

3 • Start poster contest.

This drawing contest, on subject of our choice, may be dentally related. It's a variation of our coloring competition, and again, makes for interesting and colorful wall coverage.

10 • Mail postcard from your vacation contest.

17 • Update bulletin board.

24 • Draw for No-Cavity Club 2nd quarter--Mr Zoo animal.

Don't be concerned if every topic mentioned above isn't completely clear. The purpose of reproducing part of our calendar is to exhibit our organizational **SYSTEM**. Each office should develop PR ideas consistent with its unique values, and target patient population. We are constantly adjusting, refining and adding new topics to this calendar, to keep it fresh and fun for staff and patients.

Of course, Thanksgiving, Christmas and any other special days we can think of are celebrated, and our office decorated appropriately for the events. (Connie, who works in our front office, loves to decorate. I'm happy to buy whatever she's gracious and ambitious enough to display, as it brightens the office, and adds a certain extra energy and fun.)

I'll be honest with you. While intensely meaningful to me, the following segment on smart charitable giving doesn't have much to do with marketing, at least in a direct fashion. (However, there are some definite possible marketing opportunities with the following plan that I'll point out.) I suggest you consider this as a bonus segment.

I fear being indicted for preaching here, but for those who feel compelled to "give back" for all the blessings they have received, this **system** is a wonderful idea. It can make charity easier and cheaper to implement, as well as enriching one's life, if the approach detailed is consistent with personal beliefs and values. This topic may not be of interest to everyone, and that's fine. But I believe a segment of readers will find the concepts highly helpful...maybe even inspiring.

Support Charity the Smart Way

Dentistry is a profession of givers in a nation with a heritage of caring and helping. To buttress this contention, consider that over 600,000 IRS-approved American charities exist. (And I seem to be on each one's mailing list!)

For decades I've tried to do my part, giving to carefully selected causes I felt to be of worth, trusting they were legitimate entities (being "taken" by two bogus charities of which I'm aware), dealing with increasingly more demanding recordkeeping, hoping my gifts resulted in some good, although never able to personally witness that they did.

Wouldn't it be perfect to assist worthwhile charities, while an independent third party assures they are legitimate, to receive a major tax incentive in return for one's contribution, while all the bookkeeping, tax documentation, even mailing of checks is done for you? Too good to be true? I would have agreed, until I discovered charitable gift, or donor-advised, funds.

How It Works

One may establish a charitable gift fund with various forms of assets--cash or securities--but once gifts are made to the fund, they are irrevocable. The contributed assets can be used for making grants to fund endowments, scholarships, or memorials. These funds often serve as an alternative to a private foundation, because they are less costly to establish, and easier to administer.

It is ideal to use stocks that have appreciated in value, and upon which one will owe significant taxes when they are sold, to fund a charitable account. Such equities can be sent directly to the fund, rather than selling the stocks yourself, and sending a check to the charity. Allowing the fund to sell the stock directly assures there will be no confusion (or possible IRS challenges) regarding taxes. One deducts the full value of the shares contributed (not just their initial cost) from his or her taxes the year in which the gift is made.

The fund I've used assesses no loads or fees from one's donations. The only expenses are the normal fees charged to manage mutual funds that vary from 1 percent to .45 percent, depending on one's choice of financial instruments in which to hold his or her contributions.

Once the fund is established, you select the charity and the timing of your gifts, then fill out and mail a simple form to the fund indicating the desired amount of your gift, and the name and address of the cause you wish to support. The fund verifies that you have selected an IRS-approved charity, and sends them a check, along with a letter identifying the patron, and explaining your gift (unless the donor chooses to remain anonymous). You receive statements that verify your giving according to IRS standards.

For Example

Assume you purchased shares of stock some time ago for \$2,500. While grateful the equities have appreciated to be worth \$10,000 today, you are unhappy to owe a capital gains tax on the \$7,500 profit (28 percent capital gains tax rate x \$7,500 profit = \$2,100 of taxes due) if the securities are sold.

Rather than contributing after-tax dollars (money remaining after federal, state, local, FICA and Medicare taxes are paid), you decide to gift these stocks to charity. By so doing, you avoid the \$2,100 capital gains tax and IN ADDITION, receive a tax deduction for the entire \$10,000 face value of the stocks in the year you make the gift. The dollar value of the deduction depends on one's tax bracket, which could be as high as 38 percent, providing a \$3,800 net tax savings to accompany the \$2,100 capital gains tax savings. Not bad for an initial \$2,500 investment!

Personal Value

Saving significant tax dollars and hassles on personal giving is wonderful, but the reason one contributes to charity is to help others. The money in the fund can be used to concentrate your giving, and offer significant aid to charities and organizations of your choosing. Before establishing the fund, our family used a "shotgun" approach, firing little pellets of **after-tax** charitable dollars toward most who asked. The above detailed tax advantages allow much greater giving, for the SAME net after-tax cost. Also, since employing the fund, we've chosen to focus our giving, like a high-powered rifle, to maximize its effect.

Jo and I decided to keep the money near home, and support our financially challenged school district that has been jettisoning "non-essential" programs as a floundering ship tosses cargo. We established a fine arts department that has produced plays the past three years--the first theater our high school has enjoyed for over a decade.

We also instituted a writing program that involves everyone from elementary through high-school students. Annual writing contests are held, the winning works published in a local paper, and every entry compiled in book form by a local printer for the students and parents to keep. Prizes--mainly consisting of gift certificates to a local bookstore and government savings bonds--are given to first, second and third place entries. We've also supported a track and weight training program (we bought the weights), both new to our system, and struggling to begin.

Dentistry, and the community in which we live, have blessed our family financially. Reading the winning essays, watching students (many of them patients) perform in plays--none of which would have existed if not for our support--is a rewarding source of personal satisfaction I never received from dropping a check in the mail.

I present our experience only to illustrate possible uses of donor-advised funds. There are many worthy causes desperately seeking money on a local, national and international level. I believe you'll find the process of determining which causes you'll support to be a pleasant and interesting exercise.

While we make no effort to advertise our giving, in our small community there are few secrets, and these projects reflect well on our office. I believe such endeavors enhance our bond with existing patients, and may result in new patients seeking our care...a not unpleasant side-effect.

One could easily choose to employ these charitable efforts as part of a practice marketing strategy. One could give a scholarship to a local high school graduate, perhaps someone interested in science. Such a gift is usually presented in person at an awards program--where local press coverage is almost certain--and bears the name of the dentist or practice.

Last year, Jo and I gave the largest donation to a new Big Brother, Big Sister program in our area. The director called and requested a photo of us appear in the paper. We declined, but what a wonderful "marketing tool" such a gift could be, helping others in need, while presenting one's values to the community, all in a tax-efficient manner! The opportunities to market through meaningful giving are limited only by one's imagination.

How to Begin

Fidelity was the first financial service company to sponsor a donor-advised program, having begun operations in September of 1992. Similar funds are beginning to be offered by other firms (I imagine motivated by this fund's success), but Fidelity Investments Charitable Gift Fund is the company with whom I've dealt and the only one, to my knowledge, with any significant existing track record.

Opening a Charitable Gift Fund takes only a few minutes--about like opening a checking account. There is a minimum $10,000 initial contribution, but while you deduct the entire amount from your taxes the year the gift is made (subject to deduction limits set by the IRS), you can use these contributed dollars, and the income they earn, to fund your giving for as many years as you like--even after your death.

You have a choice of four pools of funds in which you can place your money. The growth pool, which we selected, has returned an average of 15.3 percent annually since its 1992 inception. While you receive no further deductions from these earnings, the income the fund creates is reinvested to generate more assets in your account, which are available to give to worthy causes you select.

Please consult your tax adviser to see how this strategy can best work for you. You may reach Fidelity's Charitable Gift Fund by calling 1-800-682-4438 or faxing 1-617-476-7824. Ask for information on the Charitable Gift Fund, and begin supporting charity the smart way.

(The author has no interest in, nor does he receive any form of compensation from, Fidelity Investments...which is sort of a shame, now that I think about it.)

SEGMENT III

Chapter 9

Practice Building Through Comfort: Gentle, Profound, Predictable Anesthesia

We'll confine our clinical considerations, in this resource, to focusing on a subject few dentists would dispute is critical to both practice growth and attaining clinical superiority, yet one infrequently addressed. It's the art and science of gentle, profound, and predictable anesthesia.

I've written about this foundational topic before, but I feel the information is worthy of reexamination. I include it in our ongoing hygiene discussion, as obtaining anesthesia predictably and comfortably is an important step in one's efforts to enhance patient volume--critical to practice growth--whether one's objective is to implement highly profitable expanded hygiene, or just to enable one's spouse to shop in the better malls.

Also, as one enhances the level of periodontal treatment offered by his or her practice, half-mouth numbings will be performed on hygiene patients on a fairly routine basis. It's important to be able to provide this amount of anesthesia comfortably, yet skillfully and efficiently, so the least possible dosage can be employed.

I reiterate my desire to have this book serve as a stand-alone resource, containing everything relevant and requisite to outstanding, profitable hygiene. The techniques of providing ideal care, with maximum comfort, are an important portion of that quest, and mastering such skills represents huge strides in one's journey to clinical excellence and practice dominance.

Few would argue against the assertion that even the most gifted dentist can't provide his or her best treatment for a squirming, let alone screaming, patient. **If one can't numb teeth well, one can't consistently provide excellent care.** Soon this critical lack of skill won't matter, as, **if one has trouble obtaining profound anesthesia, or causes excessive discomfort when he or she injects, few patients will be coming to see you anyway!**

But don't all doctors provide "gentle, profound, and predictable anesthesia"? Not according to many of the patients I see. After I'd completed giving anesthesia, one sweet lady in her seventies told me, "That's the first shot I've gotten in my life that didn't hurt." (Seventy years is a long time to wait...for anything.)

Do you think there is a chance my newest senior friend alluded to this blessed, and for her singular, event in conversation with anyone else? Is it possible the people to whom she mentioned my pain-free technique also prefer injections that don't hurt, and would consider leaving their current dental home in search of this painless Mecca? (Just to help get you going...the answers to the above semi-rhetorical posers are "Yes" and "Yes.")

I believe most doctors assume "my shots don't hurt" (at least not much)...but start observing your patients. Do they tense, close their eyes (or occasionally kick their feet and scream)? All these behaviors could be subtle clues that things aren't as comfortable as one had hoped.

Possibly I'm unique, but I can feel the tension in a patient, as surely as if I'd grabbed a bare electric wire, and it doesn't feel good (for either of us). Their pulse becomes my pulse, and their blood pressure, mine. (Sounds like a form of aversion therapy!) And the dentist gets to experience this sensation 10 or so times a day! The patient at least only has to put up with it once.

This brings me to a second major point about anesthesia: "gentle, profound, and predictable anesthesia" can save, or at least prolong, a life...yours. Nothing in dentistry is as stressful to me as treating a patient who can "feel it," or even a patient who has psychic powers and suspects she may be about to "feel it."

I once traveled 200 miles to watch a noted endodontist ply his trade. If I assimilated any clinical gems from my odyssey--which was my journey's intent--I've long ago forgotten them. But, during the course of his day, my specialist friend incised and drained an abscess in the number 30 area for an elderly emergency patient. The procedure didn't take long, but the area was quite swollen, and this lady "felt it." When the abscess was opened, and the screaming and kicking stopped, I found myself out in the hall with sweat on my lip and a bad headache. Thank God I was only watching!

To me, the most amazing part of this whole scenario was the behavior of patients in the reception room...they were still there! Such unhappy occurrences are not good for the reputation of the profession of dentistry, or for the dentist, staff, and patients involved.

So, I hope you'll grant me these three points:

1. Treating patients without profound anesthesia, or hurting them during the injection, is stressful to everybody in the room. It's

something dentists would like to avoid, if for no other reason than saving wear and tear on our bodies and souls.

2. Treating patients who are comfortable is mandatory for dentists who wish to consistently offer the best care of which they are capable.
3. The ability to provide gentle, profound, predictable anesthesia may be the biggest practice builder in existence. (Or lack of this vital skill may have the most negative impact on a practice possible.) My years of clinical experience have allowed me to become acquainted with a lot of people whose former dentist hurt them. Most of us don't want to be the next former dentist, so let's explore how to avoid this fate.

Allow me to begin with this disclaimer: As with about everything else, I'm no expert, and possess no special "gift" for administering local anesthetic. However, the critical act of numbing teeth is an area where the playing field is even. Any dentist, of any skill level (even mine!), given sufficient motivation and concern, can learn to give painless and effective injections.

A major reason behind my unlikely practice success--as I sure don't appear to have much going for me--is I am a dentist who tries everything possible to assure the care I offer doesn't hurt. It's not so much that I'm a compassionate guy--I love to hunt and kill animals, for gosh sakes!--but I just can't stand to hurt people. That bothers me--a lot, for many days...and sleep-disturbed nights.

It should also be stated that any dentist who does give painful shots is **guilty of not doing one's best to avoid hurting another human being**. If I realized I no longer cared if I caused others pain...I'd take a long vacation and deeply reflect on just where in hell my life was going! Making a deep, almost spiritual commitment to painlessness can, for some, be the beginning of a rebirth of their practice, finances, joy and soul.

Let's continue our pattern of unabashed candor. No matter the level of the provider's concern or skill, some of what we have to do just isn't much fun. Many dental procedures are innately unpleasant (such as all types of semi-suffocating impressions, even when the material used doesn't taste like sh__!)

We make our living working in the intimate and ultra-sensitive mouth, the birthplace and epicenter of infant sensations. Some discomfort is just a portion of the profession with which all dentists must come to grips. But the awareness that I was indifferent to causing others avoidable pain would lead me to reexamine my life!

Despite my self-confessed lack of manual dexterity (my nickname is "hands-of-stone"; my baseball glove was made by U.S. Steel, etc.), I do possess a secret weapon! I have the good fortune to be terrified of needles (the sharp, pointy end of same, at least). This anxiety has given me an empathy that borders on the supernatural, and explains my selfish reasons (namely personal psychic terror) for trying so diligently not to cause any discomfort when injections are given. **Comfortable shots are mainly a product of the injector's will and attitude...and, good news, we all control our will and attitude!**

I was a terrified child, who screamed his way through every injection (while my baby sisters smiled and didn't even blink...the traitors!). It's difficult for me to comprehend that this very dread is a trait that significantly explains the success I've enjoyed in dentistry! As my grandmother often inquired, "Will wonders never cease?"

All that finally clarified to my satisfaction, I believe we have two separate subjects to address:

1. Gentle anesthesia.
2. Profound and predictable anesthesia.

Gentle:

I've often wondered, do my patients love me, or is it my nitrous oxide? I suppose, if nitrous oxide sedation were outlawed, I would have still practiced dentistry, but I try not to think about things like that. Nitrous plays such a central role in my war against dental pain that, while I feel it deserves to be mentioned first, we'll devote the entire last half of this chapter to a detailed discussion of nitrous oxide- a blessing I believe no office that desires to be the best should choose to function without.

My next best "gentle" helper is a good topical anesthetic, placed on dried tissue for about 30 seconds before injecting. I've had doctors tell me topicals don't reduce discomfort. It's easy to find out. Just inject yourself with a few drops of local (you big chicken), applying topical on one side of your cheek, and not on the other. There's no reason one should take my word for it, and this experiment should eliminate doubt as to topical's effectiveness.

I think most brands of topical work well, so I select mine primarily on the basis of smell and taste. Even the sensation of numbness before the needle, and the knowledge that the dentist is concerned enough to provide this extra care, are important practice builders when brought to the patient's attention. During the examination appointment, I explain that we numb the gums before we numb the teeth, thus most patients will feel no discomfort during the injection. Placing a small dollop of topical on the patient's tongue during this first visit is a convincing demonstration, as the entire mouth feels numb in a few seconds. This simple act of exhibiting the profound effect of topicals probably reduces our failure rate and perhaps increases case acceptance.

I always "wiggle" the tissue vigorously while placing the needle and injecting. Short of knocking the patient to the floor, I don't believe you can create too much motion. As I understand it, this concept is part of the "gate" theory of pain. If nerves are relaying a movement or pressure sensation to the brain, they can't carry the "ouch" message. Again, it has been my experience that the more exuberantly one wiggles, the less pain the patient feels--even when giving mandibular blocks.

The last point about "gentle" is the most critical: **GO SLOWLY!** One can gauge ideal injection speed by the patient's reactions. If one injects too quickly, he or she will feel the patient tense. I've watched numerous dentists give anesthetic, and they invariably inject a lot faster than I.

I don't believe it takes any additional time to inject slowly. After the fast injection, the dentist must wait for the anesthetic to take effect (and the patient's back to un-arch--"Don't treat them until their butt is back in the chair"--I guess).

Instead of stabbing, then jabbering, I always carry on a conversation, while I'm patiently and gently injecting, to help divert the patient. (If you know the patient's spouse is having an affair, mentioning the situation during the injection would be an almost perfect distraction...unless you sense the patient may be prone to violence!) At first, it's a little hard to find something to discuss at a tension-filled moment like this, but with experience and effort, this conversational diversion becomes second nature. (I have become master of the rhetorical question!) Focusing the patient's mind on **anything** other than the needle's pointy end helps.

I've had a surprising number of patients comment that they love the way I chatter on, during "the shot." I'm astonished that they realize this is a deliberate effort to distract them, but most are grateful for this "technique" that allows them to be more comfortable.

In summary, my suggestions for gentle anesthesia include:

1. Nitrous oxide, that we'll discuss in a moment.
2. Topical.
3. Spin a web of conversation. Somewhere in the middle of the monologue, give the injection.
4. Wiggle tissues vigorously throughout the entire injection process.
5. Slow injection. One can't go too slowly, or hurt too little.

Profound and Predictable:

Here I'm really not an expert, but I'd like to humbly share a few of the little things I do that help achieve complete anesthesia for my patients.

1. Occasionally upper molars, especially second and third molars, won't get numb, even for routine operative, without palatal anesthesia. (I suspect this situation is the result of a lingual root projecting unusually far into the dense palatal bone. You've probably all extracted such straddled-out monsters, usually with a significant portion of the buccal plate still attached to the roots.) When a buccal infiltration followed by a firm injection of a carpule directly into buccal bone hasn't proven effective, palatal anesthetic usually numbs the tooth almost instantly.

   THE PAD, a device invented by Dr. William E. Mason, a periodontist, has helped me give much more comfortable palatal injections. After applying topical, the instrument is used to place firm pressure directly over the palatine foramen. Because The Pad has a hole in the center, one can inject while keeping pressure constant. Patients report feeling more pressure than pain when such a system is employed. One may order

The Pad from Dr. Mason by calling 517-792-4431 or faxing 517-792-4387. One of these things will probably last a lifetime. All three dentists in our office feel The Pad is helpful.

Just before retirement, I began to use another promising technique to give comfortable palatal injects. I slipped the needle into the sulcus in the lingual center of the tooth, and slowly injected, seeing the tissue blanch as I gently applied pressure. The three times I tried this (of course, with topical and nitrous in place), the patient felt no pain.

2. To achieve anesthesia painlessly on the maxillary central incisors, I inject a full carpule over the canine, wait about a minute, then infiltrate half a carpule over the central I'm going to treat. If one goes slowly, this doesn't hurt, and the patient is usually amazed, as past injections in this sensitive area were so excruciatingly painful (from that "former" dentist).

   Once the buccal mucosa is anesthetized, one can achieve anterior palatal numbness painlessly! First, inject a few drops of anesthetic, coming from the facial direction, into the papilla on either side of the tooth one wishes to numb. The palatal tissue near the tooth will blanch.

   If one is treating a primary tooth, this buccal papilla infiltration is usually enough to achieve complete anesthesia. If not, after waiting a few seconds, one can inject directly into the blanched palatal area to augment the numbness already present. (Employing the Pad, and the Patch we'll discuss shortly, is also helpful in assuring painless anterior palatal injections.)

   I clearly recall, as a dental student, numbing a maxillary central incisor on a young man as carefully as I could.

During the injection, I'd fixed all my attention on the needle's tip. (This single point meditation was probably required due to my shaking hands!) When I completed giving anesthesia, I was horrified to discover the tears occasioned by the pain of my injection filled the EARS of my patient. This memory still disturbs me. There is no reason for anything like this to occur today, with our tiny needles and excellent technique.

3. Mandibular blocks can present significant challenges. Here are the techniques I use, reported in the sequence in which they are employed.
    a) I've used the Gow-Gates block routinely for years. It's safer and more comfortable, in my opinion. It's also simple to learn. (I believe the ADA still has a video available demonstrating this technique.)
    b) Routine mandibular block. If the patient is "jumpy" I may give both the Gow-Gates and conventional block, before I even begin a procedure. Once again, as with all blocks, I wiggle tissues vigorously throughout the injection.
    c) Buccal and mental infiltration. If I were performing multiple crowns, an extraction or molar endodontics on a new patient--or a nervous one--I might use all three of the above listed techniques before beginning a procedure. Neither infiltration is usually required for operative, and I'm not recommending them for every patient. I know it's a lot of anesthesia, and medically may not be the wisest, but I like my patients to be free of all discomfort. (No one ever says, "I think I was too well anesthetized." If they aren't completely numb, one can count on them mention-

ing it.)

d) Mandibular lingual infiltration--this I rarely need--usually just for endodontics or removal of a lower molar. The mandibular lingual bone is much thinner than the buccal plate, so lingual infiltration is more effective. One needs to bend the needle at a 45-degree angle, and employ significant pressure, to inject into this thin, tough tissue.

e) I alternate between Carbocaine and Lidocaine, as this reduces toxicity and, I believe, increases the effectiveness of the locals. **I use Carbocaine first**, as the more neutral pH makes the injection more comfortable, then re-inject with longer-acting Lidocaine, when required.

We are using **THE PATCH**, basically a strong topical anesthetic placed on an adhesive strip, more all the time. It works very well in hygiene, to allow thorough cleaning of a single sensitive area, and helps to numb the palate before an injection, or to provide adequate pain relief to place a rubber dam, seat a crown with a sub-gingival margin, remove a suture in a swollen area, etc.

I also use Marcaine for any long appointments, such as multiple crowns, or for those few but frustrating patients who seem to become profoundly numb, but whose tissues regain sensation rapidly, and for all endo and the rare extraction I perform. The duration of anesthesia is excellent, and studies show reduced postoperative soreness after Marcaine's use.

I have read about, but not used, the Stabident system. Interested dentists will have to explore this technique on their own. I will add that, were I the inventor, I would change the name. I'm a confessed needle-phobic, and I see no advantage to using the phrase "stab" in this delicate context!

I used the X-system--invented by eminent endodontist, educator and all-around good guy Dr. Kit Weathers--for about the last year of practice, and found it very effective. I made a modification of its use, sort of accidentally, that made the system even more appealing to me.

I'd ordered the system, and even **read the directions** (see how serious I am about anesthesia!). I waited until the first sensitive tooth-ALWAYS A LOWER MOLAR FOR ME--appeared. I'd spent good money (something like $30 for the introductory kit) to procure the X-system, so was ready to give it a try.

I'd already given about five injections, including buccal, mental and lingual infiltration, before resorting to the X-system, so had no need to infiltrate over the area. I placed the little osseous drill in the slow speed, got all set to cut bone...and didn't want to.

I took my syringe, with the short, stiff needle of the X-system attached, and injected forcefully to the mesial and distal of the tooth. I picked up my handpiece and **immediately** went to work. The patient was completely comfortable.

I only needed the system about 10 times that last solo year of patient care. (That means 10 days of misery were saved, for the patients, and for me. I really take it hard when I can't keep patients completely comfortable.) I always used it without the bone burr and sleeve, and it worked fine each time. I only had about 20 minutes of profound anesthesia, but that was usually enough. I'd guess the system might work even better with the drill, but I'm just such a baby! But I'll tell you this, **I'd never practice again without the X-system being available.**

You can contact Dr. Kit Weathers and his fine companions by calling 800-682-9847.

So, there are a few "nuggets" from the creek bed of my experience. Maybe dentists take this foundational skill for granted. We shouldn't. I believe taking the time to be sincerely concerned about patient comfort--and gentle, profound local anesthetic is certainly only one way among many where one can show one's commitment--is the "greatest practice builder" and one every dentist should think and talk about.

For some more recent graduates, an increase in skill or technique may be required, but for most experienced doctors, I believe achieving optimal patient comfort to be only a matter of carefully considering the benefits to them, their practice, and patients that more attention to painless local anesthesia can provide. Once the positive impact of painlessness is clearly comprehended, I believe the needed effort will be forthcoming, if only for selfish reasons of enhancing the quality of the dentist's practice and life.

For many patients, the single biggest concern of any dental appointment--more than fee, convenience, or pleasantness of the staff-is "Will this hurt?" For the true needle-phobic, little else matters. It's very possible for any caring dentist to look any patient in the eye and say, "No, it will not."

Patients today, at least in Keokuk, seem to take our profession's claim of "painless dentistry" seriously. That's great news to the offices that can fulfill their demands, but a crippling blow to those that can't. All the discussion of patient loyalty may boil down to this...most patients simply won't tolerate being hurt, even a little.

Over the years, many patients who left our practice--usually as a result of our higher fees--have returned after a single experience with a painful injection, or a procedure performed despite failure to achieve complete anesthesia. (We discussed the letter we send, welcoming all patients who leave our practice back if we can help in any way, in the previous segment.) Patients often apologize for leaving, and thank us for accepting them back. "I made a big mistake!" is a phrase often stated upon their return. Consistently numbing teeth thoroughly and painlessly gives one a tremendous competitive advantage with modern apprehensive, and often demanding, patients.

Sure, it will take a little more time and effort on the dentist's part to keep this painless promise, but if you or a loved one were the patient, wouldn't it be worth it?

Nitrous Oxide

We'll continue our discussion concerning building a deep patient base (and a highly profitable practice) by utilizing the skills that result in painlessness, with the in-depth examination of nitrous oxide I promised earlier.

Let's continue in our habitual candor. It's therapeutic, if not pleasant, to accept the fact that there are times (and for me their names are legion) when dentistry isn't much fun. It isn't fun for the patient, it isn't fun for dentists or their staff...sometimes the birds outside my office are uptight!

A plethora of events and circumstances conspire to rain unpleasantness on our tooth parade, but I believe we can agree that the two most common and severe storm fronts to rock our small office worlds fall under the general headings of **anxiety and pain**.

Fortunately, we have the capability to greatly subdue our profession's two implacable foes. Dr. Horace Wells unveiled this boon in 1844--shortly before I entered the profession--and it has been undergoing refinement ever since. I refer, of course, to nitrous oxide...my old friend laughing gas.

I fancy myself a scientist (however, I also believe I'm funny and good company...), so the data that follows will be in the form of a classic pro-con discussion concerning the features, benefits and drawbacks of nitrous. But allow me to advise you, the overriding tenor of my comments will take the form of a paean--a hymn of praise--to the wonders of this fine adjunct to our difficult profession.

I retain hazy memories of my pre-nitrous days. These experiences occurred during dental school, and two years of military service. But nitrous and I began private practice simultaneously in 1974, and we have been compatriots ever since.

We will begin our discussion by detailing the **numerous benefits** of nitrous. Soon enough, as with all things, we'll confront the problems that exist.

As we've discussed, perhaps the single most essential ingredient to private practice success is the proficiency of the dentist in consistently providing quality care with **COMFORT**. Expanded hygiene is moot if one doesn't possess this ability, as nothing will keep most patients whom you've hurt in your practice.

For the great majority of patients, comfort (that must be both emotional and physical) can best be achieved by your exhibiting concern and gentleness, and by demonstrating the ability to provide complete, consistent and painless anesthesia. Nitrous is an invaluable ally in the pursuit of these essential goals.

Nitrous provides both a sedative, or calming, and analgesic, or pain-reducing, effect. Thus nitrous relaxes patients at the usually anxious moment of injection, as well as throughout the remainder of their care, while simultaneously elevating their pain threshold.

Nitrous, in combination with a good topical, and a highly skilled, feather-gentle, slower-than-a-glacier injection technique, allows virtually every delivery of local anesthetic to be given painlessly.

If you are a brave person, you may have trouble grasping this concept, but as a self-confessed and still-practicing needle-phobic, allow me to assure you once again that, to many of us quivery humans, the availability of painless injections is an **extremely** important issue-of surpassing more intimate concern than the Social Security crisis, the national debt, or nuclear disarmament.

Some adults--about half in my practice--prefer not to use nitrous. A few others use it only during injections, then ask us to remove it altogether, or to greatly reduce their level of sedation once anesthetic has been administered. The majority who use nitrous oxide find they are much more comfortable remaining within the relaxing influence of these soothing gases during their entire dental experience. Whatever their desire, I'm happy to comply with our patients' every wish, as our prime objective is to maximize their comfort during the course of care.

As helpful as nitrous proves to be when administering adult anesthetic, **nitrous oxide is close to a miracle for the treatment of primary teeth**. I haven't been forced to give local anesthetic to complete restorations on primary teeth for several decades, even for deeper fillings.

I vividly recall the first time I used only nitrous to restore primary teeth. On that fateful day, very early in my career, necessity was indeed the mother of invention. My patient was tiny, barely 2 years old, with classic early baby-bottle syndrome caries. I had started nitrous oxide and already applied topical. As I sat with syringe in hand, I simply couldn't bring myself to inject the maxillary anterior region on this tiny child. (I suspect I still had much to learn regarding painless injections at this tyro stage of professional maturation.)

The anterior decay was fairly superficial, so I decided to attempt treatment without anesthetic. (I felt a pedodontic referral of this 20-pound youngster with multiple caries to be imminent, so saw no reason to put the patient or me through the trauma of injections.)

To my amazement, we restored four areas of decay without a whimper or wiggly from our Lilliputian patient. During that experience, my world irrevocably changed, and for the better.

The advantages of not needing local for primary teeth are many and obvious. No one likes injections--not patients, not parents, not doctors--no matter how hard we attempt to make them comfortable. The fear of pain and of needles, the terror of a child whose face is "frozen stiff" (adults know the feeling will eventually leave, but a 3-year-old doesn't), the possibilities of lip biting, accidental inter-venous injection and overdose, paraesthesia--are all concerns I can live very well without.

Using nitrous alone--with no local anesthetic--primary teeth can be restored without discomfort, and the relaxing sensation is especially pleasant for children. **Virtually every child we treat is enthusiastic and enjoys the dental experience**. Over the years, many youngsters have expressed disappointment that they had no more decay to be restored!!!! In stark contrast, I've never restored a single permanent tooth where I felt the patient had a wonderful time, and regretted needing no additional treatment. (Of course, the adults also get the bill.)

In the past, the "rubber" smell of the nosepieces was objectionable to some kids, and presented a barrier to getting them to first use nitrous. (Once kids experience the pleasant sensation, the nosepiece is no longer a concern.) Agreeably scented nasal hoods have eliminated that problem. I simply ask a child to smell the bubble gum in our magic nose. (My favorite flavor--of many available--for kids.)

Just a breath or two of "bubble gum," and they begin to visibly relax. Today's nosepieces not only come in delicious scents, but are soft, comfortable, well-fitting and available in three sizes--so little gas leaks into the patient's eyes, and the air dental team members breathe.

The best nasal hoods I've used, the softest and most pleasant-smelling, come from the ACCUTRON company. You may reach these nitrous specialists by calling 800-531-2221.

At the beginning of treatment, the caregiver must be certain kids are breathing through the nose. Some nervous kids will "sneak" air from the side of their mouths. I remind them to breathe through the bubble-gum nose, and sometimes gently lay a finger on their lips, to be certain they comply. (You'll clearly note any attempt to mouth-breathe, and can reinforce nasal inhalation.) Nitrous onset is so fast you can begin care within one or two minutes of the first breath--much quicker than is possible using local anesthetic.

Lest you think I have some unique hypnotic ability which allows me alone to perform these feats of seeming legerdemain--or that perhaps my breath induced comatose states--all the dentists who have associated in my office have also routinely restored primary teeth without using local anesthetic.

Certainly, nitrous would be invaluable to my office if only for the above stated uses. But nitrous just keeps on giving. It eliminates the gag reflex in almost all patients, while retaining the protective cough reflex. I offered orthodontic and orthopedic care, so we took frequent study models on kids. If they gagged when the tray was tried in, my assistants asked me to start nitrous oxide before attempting the alginate impression. Nitrous was also helpful for my final impressions on fixed and removable prosthetic patients with gagging tendencies. Nitrous was also a big help--reducing anxiety, increasing comfort, decreasing salivary flow and tongue mobility--when placing a fixed orthodontic appliance.

Because nitrous reduces patients' salivary flow and tongue mobility, my life was made decidedly more pleasant, and consistently offering my best possible care became easier and more predictable.

This benefit is particularly critical when placing sealants (almost all of ours are placed in hygiene), as a dry field is the difference between success and failure with this procedure.

The analgesic effect seems more pronounced on soft tissue, making prophys more comfortable, thus reducing your patient's and hygienist's stress, and giving your comfortable practice a PR boost. As mentioned, nitrous is plumbed to our every operatory, including the two rooms dedicated to hygiene. The more advanced periodontal care one offers, the more benefit nitrous in the hygiene area will provide. Treating periodontal disease is demanding. Even the gentle and skillful Melissa is grateful for all the help she can get.

Mobile primary teeth can be simply, safely and comfortably removed using just nitrous and topical anesthetic. Other uncomfortable, yet not really painful procedures, such as suture removal, dry socket treatment or crown seating, can be done much more pleasantly, and without local, by using nitrous oxide.

But it is time to approach the dark side. The grim news: nitrous oxide is not a panacea. Certain situations and patients exist where using nitrous is contraindicated.

There is some debate concerning the safety of using nitrous during pregnancy. I choose **never** to offer it to pregnant patients. I also don't use nitrous on patients with a history of drug or alcohol abuse, fearing the sensation may trigger a renewal of their addiction.

If patients can't breathe through their nose, due to a cold or allergies, nitrous can't help us. (I reschedule kids unable to breathe through their nose, rather than treat them with local.) Claustrophobics can't stand to have the nose covered, and some people find the nitrous oxide sensation to be unpleasant. (Virtually no kids object to the "floaty" feeling.)

Nitrous is contraindicated for patients with chronic obstructive pulmonary diseases, such as emphysema, severe chronic bronchitis and tuberculosis. This entire list of patients for whom nitrous oxide isn't available accounts for less than 5 percent of the people I treat.

There are no known allergies to nitrous oxide, and the gas is not irritating to the respiratory system (i.e., causes no coughing). Because nitrous is not absorbed by the blood, but leaves the body quickly through the lungs, no organ system must break the drug down to excrete it. Most patients feel no lingering effects of nitrous after the five minutes of pure oxygen I give them while I am completing the last portion of that day's treatment.

The most common nitrous oxide side effect is nausea and vomiting. This occurs most frequently with children, and results from too much gas, for too long a period of time. Dentists need to learn to observe their patients for signs they are too sleepy, then reduce the gas level accordingly. (Nitrous is simple and safe--much more so than local anesthetic--but as with everything else entailing people, there is some technique involved in its use.) I haven't had a patient vomit while on nitrous for many years.

Nitrous Dosage

I personally begin all kids on 5 liters of oxygen and 4 liters of nitrous. On rare occasions, I need to increase the nitrous oxide to 5 liters to get the desired effect, but I never go above the 50 percent level for any patient. (Higher amounts than this exceed my personal comfort zone.) If a child is too sleepy--you'll see them begin to nod off--reducing the nitrous to 3 liters invariably solves the problem.

I begin most adults on 5 liters of oxygen and 3 liters of nitrous. While nitrous oxide acts as an analgesic on primary teeth, one benefits mostly from the sedative effect on adults (we must still establish profound local anesthetic to treat all permanent teeth, no matter what the patient's age), so lower doses are adequate for our purpose.

I find the level of nitrous needed to achieve our desired relaxation on adults varies from 1 to 5 liters, with 90 percent of patients feeling maximum comfort between 2 and 3 liters.

The first time nitrous is being used on an adult (begun, as I've stated, at 5 liters oxygen, 3 liters nitrous), I ask patients to tell me immediately if they feel uncomfortably drowsy, and I adjust the nitrous oxide level down. If, two minutes after the nosepiece's placement, a patient feels no effect, I increase the nitrous level. Once we have identified a particular patient's ideal comfort zone, I note this nitrous dosage on their chart, and use that level at every subsequent visit.

Some medical conditions are aided by using nitrous. Room air has a 20.9 percent oxygen concentration. When using nitrous, I never give less than 50 percent oxygen, so for any patient where enhanced oxygen flow is beneficial--such as angina and cardiac sufferers--nitrous is helpful.

Nitrous acts as a muscle relaxant, and reduces the stress and discomfort of dental care for patients with tender TMJs, or even back pain sufferers.

There are concerns about possible consequences to the health of staff members exposed to trace nitrous oxide in the operatories. The studies available on this topic are somewhat confusing. Many deal with hospital operating rooms where other gases are used in combination with nitrous. Some dental studies took place without scavengers being part of the systems evaluated.

Let me stress that scavengers--which greatly reduce the level of nitrous oxide in operatories--should always be a part of any nitrous system. Rooms should be well ventilated. Working with a rubber dam reduces staff nitrous exposure, and patients should be limited in their talking--all efforts that reduce trace gas levels within treatment areas.

The medical concerns for staff members exposed frequently to trace amounts of nitrous include reduced fertility, possibly greater chance of spontaneous abortion, and some potential tendency to increased liver and kidney problems.

I have reviewed all available studies concerning dangers to staff from trace nitrous oxide. I'm not sure a definitive answer has been reached, but when nitrous is used properly, as we've just described, I am not personally concerned about trace nitrous health risks. (Had I any anxiety, I wouldn't have exposed myself to the gas for 26 years. However, considering the shape I'm in, that statement is far to the left of a ringing endorsement!)

Nitrous oxide recreational use and abuse is a problem limited almost entirely to doctors, due to their easy access. Prolonged use of nitrous oxide at very high levels will lead to neurological symptoms akin to those seen with multiple sclerosis. Nitrous oxide is a drug, and should never be used for social reasons.

The cost of installing a system can also be a barrier to using nitrous. A portable unit can be obtained for around $3,000, but I believe those who purchase such a system will find the inconvenience of dragging it around will limit their use of nitrous. (I believe I could have one portable unit available, practice with it for a year, and never once have it be in the room where I wanted it. I don't mean to brag, I just have a gift that way!)

Under ACCUTRON's (mentioned previously when we discussed their excellent nasal hoods) standard terms, an operatory can be set up with nitrous for around $700. (Think a single crown, maybe with buildup.) Often dental meeting specials will allow a system to be purchased at a significant discount, sometimes up to 50 percent off listed price. ACCUTRON seems to make a particularly diligent effort to facilitate the beginning practice's ability to afford an excellent nitrous system.

There are two advantages to nitrous which make it a value to me, at almost any price. The first is the reduction in stress and distress for my patients its use provides. This enhanced comfort greatly decreases the tension inherent in providing care for me (a fragile creature) and my staff.

Certainly, the quality of my dental work is enhanced by working on complacent, relaxed patients with reduced gag reflex, less salivary flow and tongue mobility--and I need every bit of help I can get! Nitrous even makes my jokes funny! (Or at least it helps. Some of my jokes would require divine intervention to work. At least I enjoy telling them, so someone's having fun!)

The second overwhelming advantage of nitrous oxide is in the realm of practice enhancement. I have no objections to those who assess a separate fee to cover the expense of administering nitrous, but I don't charge patients who choose to use nitrous. (In fact, it helps so much in treatment, I'd pay some people to use it!) Within a service industry, time is one's most vital and precious commodity. Nitrous saves me lots of time, so out-of-pocket expense has never concerned me.

Remember, it isn't your Yellow Pages, direct mail campaign, fancy office or even oh-so-tight margins that build a thriving dental practice. It is your patients bragging to their friends and loved ones that "My dentist doesn't hurt me!" Creating this reputation within the community is of much greater value to me than any revenue forthcoming from a nitrous fee (which might limit its use) could possibly be.

Not only is the ability to offer painless treatment the ultimate practice builder, but nothing can give me greater satisfaction than knowing I am able to provide optimal care in the most comfortable possible manner--especially for children.

I have a dream. It is to live in a world where the words "I hate dentists!" are never spoken. Nitrous is one extremely significant influence that moves my dream closer to reality.

I'm honestly baffled that nitrous isn't used every day, in every dental office. I hope the information shared in this chapter enhances dentistry's ability to provide better care--periodontal or restorative--in a more comfortable and caring environment.

SEGMENT IV

Chapter 10

Practice Enhancement Through Behavioral Mastery

Let's transition from material and techniques that enhance one's ability to provide optimal dental care in maximum comfort, **to the most vital ingredient of practice success...MASTERING THE SKILLS REQUIRED TO EFFECTIVELY AND CONSISTENTLY MODIFY PATIENTS' BEHAVIORS.**

As we discuss these essential abilities, with an emphasis on periodontal care (I'd be certain to share at least portions of the following material with all team members involved in your hygiene department), be aware that we are dealing with universal truths. These powerful concepts, when comprehended and implemented, can augment one's ability to relate to anyone, for any reason.

The attributes inherent within these talents can be implemented to improve collections, decrease failed appointments, increase case acceptance rates, achieve better results from one's chart audit efforts, etc. They can also be employed to improve communication effectiveness, and thus relationships, with patients, staff and loved ones. The ability to become involved in meaningful and lasting affiliations is imperative to achieving joy in all venues of existence.

Behavioral masters (who understand and consistently employ refined methods, such as these we are about to examine) are those somewhat puzzling, but blessed, people who can make us do what they desire--even if that's not what we think we want to do--and yet we find ourselves delighted to carry out their wishes! (I do whatever my wife asks...but that's out of fear. An entirely different, if at least as effective, dynamic.) So let's begin our efforts to understand the powerful techniques they employ.

The Art of Successful Communication

Have you ever just sat, at the end of your day, and pondered? At 11 this morning, Ms. Smith cancelled her appointment to begin periodontal care...again. Neither you, nor any other staff member, was surprised. But her problems are severe, and rapidly getting worse. Damn cigarettes. She's already having pain from recurrent periodontal abscesses.

During the examination and consultation appointments, you discussed her x-rays, and insisted she watch seeping blood and pus as you spot-probed. After full-mouth pocket charting, you personally reviewed her oral hygiene, gave her educational pamphlets, stressed the urgency of her condition--the works! You gave it your all because her problems are severe, and you really care.

But even as you labored--to explain, educate, motivate--you knew. Even as you spoke, a part of you sensed the message wasn't getting through. What could you have done? Could someone else have been more effective? The stakes are high...Ms. Smith's teeth. No well-informed and thinking person would choose to lose them! There must be some way to reach her.

I believe most dentists would agree that effective communication is **the essential ingredient in case acceptance**. Unless we get our patients to understand and embrace the course of treatment we know to be ideal for their individual needs, no matter how great our knowledge and skill, we can do nothing to help them.

I'm sure every reader has shared some version of the frustrations described in the above scenario. To me, the disappointment seems greater for periodontal problems, as treatment is relatively quick and inexpensive, and the consequences of failing to accept care-from teeth lost, to serious systemic health damage--so starkly disastrous.

Some patients hear your words and respond. They accept responsibility for their problems and enter into treatment willingly, even eagerly. They keep appointments, and diligently perform recommended home care. Their oral health, sense of peace and quality of life improve.

Others listen politely...but the light of understanding and enthusiasm is missing from their eyes. Perceptive dentists realize when they are failing to influence their patient. They are apprehensive that critical dental needs may go unmet, and aren't shocked when appointments are cancelled or failed. Yet, you've given the same basic information to both accepting and rejecting groups. Why this dramatic difference in the messages' reception and outcome?

Understanding the <u>fundamentals of human relationships</u> is essential to success, no matter what your chosen field. Without access to some form of effective communication, it's impossible to create the positive affiliations that lead to trust. Many books have been written concerning communication skills. The art of first impressions, understanding body language, neuro-linguistic programming, transactional analysis, and too many additional facets of human interaction to mention have been analyzed in exquisite detail. Great value exists in all these disciplines, but we will limit our discussion to what I believe is the most simply understood and easily improvable facet of communication ...verbal skills.

There are four primary ways by which humans process the words we hear. No one technique is superior or inferior. Each mode contains both strengths and weaknesses. The four types merely describe the varied manners in which humans relate to the world. While all of us use each of these methods, everyone has a strong tendency to favor one or two modes.

It is naive, at best, to assume the same verbal communication approach will work equally well with each of the four basic personality types. The presentation dentists repeatedly deliver to their patients is **often based on the doctor's primary personality orientation, and thus will be optimally successful with approximately one-fourth of one's audience.**

Few dentists are pleased if their urgent oral health message is accepted by a mere 25 percent of patients, and few can afford such dismal case acceptance rates. (I hope all of you monitor case acceptance--the percentage of recommended care accepted. If you don't, you may be surprised, even shocked--as I was when I first measured this critical factor--by the low compliance rate of one's patients. But such a dismaying surprise might be the emotional key to drive one to work harder to improve this vital area. Few things can so powerfully enhance a practice as significantly increasing patient acceptance of offered care.)

Let's discuss these four basic personality types. As we do, determine into which group you predominantly fall. As you consider this information, you'll find yourself identifying specific patients within each segment. Often you'll remember these patients due to the easily recalled frustration of never being able to really reach them. Think also about members of your team, your family and loved ones. Can you identify by what method each of them accesses information?

The Four Types

1. CONTROLLERS or DIRECTORS are people who have to be in charge. They are strong-willed, decisive, direct in their approach and tend to be domineering. They make quick decisions based on what is best for them, and care little how it influences others. They are interested in results, not emotions. They are willing risk-takers.

These people are always in a hurry. They want the straight facts, then will quickly decide on a course of action. If you explain every detail of your proposed treatment, you'll drive them away. (This is your author, in spades! Give me the basics, then get the hell out of my way!)

2. ANALYZERS or ENGINEERS are people who must have all the data before reaching a decision. They will desire every bit of information concerning their oral health problem available, and often request more.

If you try to rush them into a decision, they will become frustrated. They are unemotional, detail-oriented, and proceed with decisions slowly, methodically. They are definitely not risk-takers.

3. PROMOTERS or CHEERLEADERS look at the big picture and don't sweat the details. They are fun-loving folks, often storytellers. They make decisions quickly, frequently without benefit of all the facts.

They tend to be self-centered, to live for the moment, and are enjoyable to be around. They are often most concerned with appearance, and are definitely risk-takers. They have no interest in the details of their problems or treatment, and will be turned off by such a discussion.

4. SUPPORTERS or HELPERS are reluctant to make decisions. They work well with others, exhibiting tremendous concern for people's feelings. They are very anxious concerning how their actions affect others, and are intensely uncomfortable with conflict.

They go along with others' decisions easily, and are excellent workers. Strongly encouraging them to accept the care you know to be ideal will be very effective with this group.

Now that we have established a basic understanding of the four predominant ways in which people process verbal information, let's consider how we can use this knowledge to improve our effectiveness with patients.

Understanding this data is helpful in myriad ways. But, since the primary focus of this book is on periodontal care, I will suggest an ideal strategy for each group that will allow them to understand and accept a needed soft tissue treatment course. We'll also briefly observe how a similar basic approach could be employed to reinforce oral hygiene and regular re-care appointments. (These concepts are equally valid when presenting full mouth reconstruction, or any other needed treatment.)

The first step toward enhancing our communication effectiveness is to precisely identify the basic type with which we are dealing, using the descriptions just provided. No treatment should ever be recommended until the dentist is familiar enough with his or her patient to clearly distinguish the governing personality category.

Once this critical step is accomplished, one can employ his or her perception of how the patient processes data to tailor one's approach ideally to match the other's unique understanding. By employing this discernment, one can learn to almost instantly "speak every patient's language."

The EXECUTIVE type is very busy. They are always in a hurry, are upset if you're running even a few minutes behind, and have a tendency to cancel appointments due to changes in their schedule. Let's eavesdrop on a snatch of conversation with one such individual.

"Mr. Executive, I'm very troubled about the condition of your gums."

"Oh? What **facts** concern you?"

"Please look in this mirror. (Or watch the intra-oral camera, if available.) See these spaces, or pockets, along the necks of the teeth? They are getting deeper. Notice the blood seeping from some of the places I've touched?"

"Yes, I see what you mean. Doesn't look good. What can we do?"

"The most ***effective approach*** *would be a deeper cleaning, numbing your gums to make it comfortable for you."*

"How long does that take?"

"In your case, we could do all of the treatment in two additional visits."

"If that's what I need, let's get it scheduled."

There remains one last critical bit of information. At this point, SHUT UP AND SCHEDULE. This guy's made a decision, and he's done talking. He has no interest in the details. Tell him what he needs, how it can best be accomplished, and get on with it!

If your concern is improving these patients' oral hygiene, or getting them to be more faithful in their re-care appointments, stress how their compliance will be most efficient, thus saving them time and money, while enhancing final results.

Our ENGINEER type never misses an appointment, and is never late. She is diligent with home care, but her tissues still don't look as healthy as you'd like.

> *"Ms. Engineer, I'm very concerned with the condition of your gums. It seems the routine things we're trying just aren't* ***working effectively****. We're not getting the response we need to see."*
>
> "What's wrong?"

Finally, you have a chance to display all of the erudition you've gleaned from years of professional education. You can also get out a copy of each of those somewhat dusty handouts on periodontal disease. This patient will want every detail.

After a lengthy discussion, she will probably wish to think things over. Make a note to call her in a week. Ask if she has any more questions, and have some time available to visit, as she will. **Don't pressure these patients**. Engineer types will reach a decision, but only when they are ready.

When reinforcing the need for oral hygiene or regular re-care, your approach will be the same: Provide lots of facts, answer their questions, then wait patiently for them to digest all the information and reach a comfortable decision.

The CHEERLEADER will undoubtedly be one of your favorite patients. They are fun to be around, always ready to share an amusing story. They aren't, however, very reliable. They forget, fail, or are late to appointments frequently. Their oral hygiene efforts tend to be sporadic.

"Ms. Cheerleader, I'm very concerned about the health of your gums."

"What's wrong?"

"Look in this mirror (intra-oral camera screen). See how red, swollen and ***unattractive*** *these gum tissues look."*

"Oh my goodness, yes! They are all swollen. What can we do! The poor things just look awful!!"

"With proper care, we can have those gums as pink, firm, and healthy as they looked when you were a teenager."

"Really? Then let's do it!"

Once again, it's time for that critical step. SHUT UP AND SCHEDULE. You can provide additional information as you proceed with treatment, but this person wants more attractive gums, and she wants them badly. Grant her wish!

With the need for oral hygiene and regular re-care--you guessed it--appeal to how much healthier and more attractive the patient will appear with coral-pink, youthful gingival tissues. Have fun with these enjoyable folks, just emphasize the critical importance of their keeping all time commitments with you, and don't bore them to death with details.

MR. HELPER is a good patient. Not a real entertaining individual, but he never misses an appointment, or is even late. He makes a real effort to comply with your oral hygiene recommendations, even though he's a smoker.

"Mr. Helper, I'm really troubled about the condition of your gums."

> Concern clouds his face as you demonstrate what worries you with mirror or camera. "What can I do?"
> *"I'll **detail a precise course of action for you**. If you do exactly as I tell you, I'm confident that, **working together**, we can improve your oral health."*

To enhance regular re-care and oral hygiene compliance, you again prescribe a very specific course of action, and stress the two of you working as a team. These people want to make you happy, and it's reassuring to them to be given a specific, concise set of directions, as uncertainty makes them nervous.

Why go to all of this trouble? Isn't it enough to do your job and tell people the truth? Let's examine a few of the advantages inherent in identifying primary relational types, and thus improving one's communication effectiveness.

With improved communication ability, not only does the acceptance of needed care increase, but so does the APPRECIATION OF PATIENTS FOR WHAT THE DENTIST DOES. When one makes the effort to couch communications in their terms, patients feel **listened to and understood**. (And these are very pleasant feelings to have!) Because of this, they perceive the provider to be a special, insightful person. As an additional bonus, your frustration level will decrease, as it's more fun working with patients who understand and enthusiastically accept care they know to be best for them.

Of course, your clinical success rate will be much greater, now that you and your patients understand each other, and are working as a team toward a mutually understood and appreciated goal. For example, getting patients to comprehend their problem, and thus become personally committed to ideal home maintenance and re-care, is THE

KEY to successful periodontal care.

The practice's income increases, as more treatment is provided. If you compensate your hygienist by commission (as I feel every hygienist should be paid), he or she will be rewarded for greater case acceptance with an instant pay increase. (A wonderful example of capitalism at its finest!)

I believe the biggest benefit inherent from enhanced communication skills is intensified personal growth. As your team's verbal skills improve, your patients, co-workers, friends and family will perceive each of you differently. It's even easier to relate to strangers at a party using this information.

I realize this is but a thumbnail sketch of this vital topic....But with awareness and practice you'll find these skills soon becoming second nature. As a well-deserved reward for your efforts, you'll discover the world is filled with interesting people whom you can understand, relate to, enjoy and provide with optimal dental treatment.

How to Exhibit Mastery in Times of Conflict

We now have attained at least a cursory understanding of basic behavioral types. This is information most of us are exposed to, from time to time, but few ever bother to implement thoughtfully (the exception being the ultra-successful). Let's build upon this bedrock, by considering how a team can continue to work effectively, even during those periods when "the stuff done hit the fan."

Most skilled dental team members can function beautifully when the day runs smoothly, the office atmosphere is peaceful and productive. But as surely as in every life a little rain must fall, conflict will appear, even within the most sophisticated and patient-friendly practices.

I've heard MASTERY defined as "the art of exhibiting excellence under pressure." It's the times of tension that separate the best from the rest. Developing the ability to consistently deal with unavoidable strife in a calm, confident and positive manner--behavioral mastery--will augment one's chances of achieving the level of professional success, peace of mind and happiness all desire.

Office problems assume many forms, but most would agree that conflict with patients is a classic no-win situation. Even if you are "right," you will be tried and found guilty in the patient's court of opinion, from which no appeal is possible. An upset patient might not return for needed care, certainly won't refer, may disparage the practice within the community, or even seek legal redress.

If one agrees it's impossible to win such confrontations, it behooves one to consider the **ideal manner in which to approach conflicts** to assure the best possible outcomes. Let's consider a concise, four-step formula that will allow all who understand this plan to face contention with proficiency and aplomb.

Four Steps to Conflict Mastery

1. **LISTEN AND AGREE!** When faced with any form of conflict, the first step toward positive resolution is to **carefully LISTEN to the complaint, and AGREE with the complainer**. Show by body language and brief verbal feedback that you sympathize with his problem and are on his side

   Here's the hard part. To do this, one must stifle the natural urge to justify oneself mentally and verbally, and make a determined effort to focus--not on one's raging defensive internal dialog and pressing need to respond--but on hearing and understanding the unhappy person's diatribe. Establish how disappointed you are that he is disturbed. When patients are displeased, I am saddened, and stating, "I'm terribly sorry you're upset" is NOT an admission of guilt.

2. Remain on the patient's side. This is the key to draining energy from even the most vociferous complainer. It's difficult to continue protesting with one who keeps agreeing with your every statement. **Don't leap to a possible solution**, in an understandable, but ill-advised effort to forestall further criticism. Allow the patient every opportunity to vent both facts and emotions completely. An infected wound must be thoroughly drained to heal cleanly.
3. IMMEDIATELY accept full responsibility for the problem. This doesn't mean you've caused the problem. Rather, it assures the unhappy party that you possess the necessary INTEGRITY AND PERSONAL POWER to set things right. There's an overabundant supply of "it's not my fault" within our current culture. Consider...when you are faced with a problem, is it excuses you desire? Or do you long for a White Knight to appear, assume full accountability, and set things right? Just the act of someone unreservedly embracing responsibility is comforting to the person with a problem. And possessing the courage to directly face unpleasant situations is the mark of a mature person...a champion.
4. Co-develop a plan of action. Once you and the patient are clearly on the same side of the issue, and his emotional energy has been released, calmly co-develop a plan to deal with the situation in a manner acceptable to both parties.

For Example

Let's consider a hygiene example--since that is the topic of this book--to illustrate how to best achieve our primary objective of ideal conflict resolution. But understand that the information we are sharing is viable for any form of contention, whether it be personal or professional.

Mr. Entrepreneur may be a lovely person, but he is far from an ideal patient. Although he (sort of) accepted the soft tissue management program your office suggested four years ago, he has refused to buy the oral hygiene instrument you have repeatedly recommended ("Just a damn expensive toothbrush!"), and has cancelled, failed and rescheduled so often that the suggested three-month recalls have become closer to six-month intervals.

(By now, you've positively identified this patient's basic personality type...right? Remember, knowledge doesn't lead to wisdom until it is acted upon, so start employing the potential erudition your mind is assimilating at every opportunity.)

He is a heavy smoker and difficult to care for clinically, due to extreme anxiety, a strong gag reflex and sensitive teeth (not to mention breath that would gag a garbage collector!).

It had been seven months--not the three-month interval suggested--since his last visit. He strode into the operatory today, 10 minutes late, loosened his tie and advised you he had to be in a meeting within the hour. A quick probing revealed generally increased pocket depths, heavy bleeding, areas of purulent exudate and increased mobility. The routine maintenance that had been scheduled is not the solution to these profound problems. It's time to forthrightly address this patient's declining oral health.

There are three critical steps that will optimize the delivery of any important message:

a) Make firm, direct eye contact with the party to whom you are speaking.

b) Address them by an appropriate name.

c) Initiate some form of physical contact.

You upright the patient's chair, reach out and lightly touch his forearm, look him unwaveringly in the eye, call him by name and reveal these findings. You explain their significance--possibly aided by a mirror or intra-oral camera--and suggest referral to a periodontal specialist would be in his best interests.

"Are you telling me that all the time and hard-earned money I've invested in treating my gum problems in your office have been wasted!? And now you want another dentist--one I don't even know--to take over my care? What in hell is wrong with you people?"

A one-sided dialog continues in this manner. It's difficult to hear such statements when you absolutely know you've done your best. Hundreds of possible rebuttals--all justified, some amusing, some obscene--have raced through your mind. To be so vilified may be inequitable, but any show of defensiveness on your behalf will only serve to intensify resistance. However, **behavioral mastery** consists of excelling in just such unfair and unpleasant situations.

You LISTEN calmly, patiently, maintaining eye contact (no guilty glances at the floor), providing feedback by nodding understanding and trying to slip in an "I see" when Mr. E pauses to catch his by now ragged breath.

When he seems to have run down, you state quietly and deliberately how sorry you are that the most conservative approach to his problems--the one you'd try first for your or a loved one's care--has not been successful, despite your best efforts.

Inform him you'll continue to do all within your power to help maximize his oral health, but that additional assistance is now required. (You might add that dentistry knows much more about and has more possible treatments for his problem today than it did even a few years ago.)

In the situation we've described, it's easy to take the road more traveled. To officiously state that due to missed appointments (which you can by-God document!), continued smoking and poor oral hygiene, your best efforts have had little chance of success. The point being, it's not your fault! These statements would all be true, but **FIXING THE BLAME DOESN'T FIX THE PROBLEM!**

When everyone's emotions (you may well be upset too by this unfair attack) are clearly under control, and not a moment before, it is time to co-develop a plan of action. Assure Mr. E that he won't be abandoned. Your office will continue to support him, and to help resolve his problems in the best possible manner. Explain that, with his permission, an appointment will be made with the periodontist, a map to her office provided, and needed x-rays and other information sent. Since this periodontist's usual routine is to alternate re-care visits with the referring office, you'll still be able to monitor progress, answer questions and provide help in any way conceivable. (Oh goody! Lucky you!)

No one--no matter how behaviorally skilled--can control the actions of another. Nothing you say or do can guarantee Mr. E will be satisfied. But choosing this adept pattern of action can assure you of enjoying an awareness that you have continued to do your utmost behaviorally for this patient, just as you have clinically. The anger and anxiety that might have troubled you for days, had this predicament erupted into direct confrontation, will be replaced by the tranquility that accompanies the knowledge one has done his or her best under this most trying of circumstances.

Let me again stress that I believe the behaviors we've considered deal with UNIVERSAL PRINCIPLES of human deportment, applicable in any situation involving conflict, whether the other party is one's boss, co-worker, friend or family member. As with any skill, it will take time and effort to perfect such conduct. But even making the effort to move from reaction toward proactive mastery will reward one with an enhanced sense of serenity and well-being, even in the most trying times of conflict. (And such peace of mind is essential, at least to my well-being.)

After providing this powerful, but somewhat generic description of dealing with conflict, allow me to reach into my bag of personal experiences labeled "Nightmare," to offer another example of how best to deal with difficult situations and people.

Waltzing Brunnhilde

I was reviewing records before our normal morning huddle, looking forward to a pleasant and productive day (one must not lose hope!), when I noticed BRUNNHILDE's name on my schedule. Since I was semi-retired and treated patients only three days a month, it had been years since Broomy and I had last "crossed swords," but the name still caused a spasm in my gut--not a pleasant sensation--especially at 7 a.m. The scheduled treatment was for an MODF amalgam, a puzzler since I rarely placed fillings, and certainly not on teeth obviously requiring a crown.

I anxiously scanned our most recent computer notes. Broomy had appeared for her routine hygiene appointment about a week ago. She was complaining of sensitivity in the area of tooth number 30. When advised the aged filling had fractured, and the tooth required treatment, she became upset and refused to allow her periodontal care to be completed.

My associate had refused to schedule her to place this restoration. This was the first adult patient he had declined to treat in the 10 years we'd worked together. The notes stated Broomy wouldn't listen to my staff member's discussion of the need for a crown, and declined even to look at the intra-oral photo that had been taken. She demanded an appointment with me to replace "his filling," then stormed from the office.

During our morning huddle and clearing I heard the long version of Broomy's last visit from several staff, recounted as eagerly and vividly as one might describe a gory wreck on the freeway. She'd had a colorful and memorable dental visit, amusing only to those fortunate souls who hadn't been forced to deal with her directly.

I tried hard not to let concerns about her approaching appointment ruin my day. Broomy was scheduled at 4 p.m., when I would be fatigued, and the office usually very busy. Maybe she'd cancel or fail...but I knew, whatever her shortcomings, that Broomy was as predictable as morning breath. The odds of her not appearing were about the same as my getting good news on April 15th.

This patient had advanced periodontal problems, but adamantly refused a specialist referral, while keeping her three-month hygiene appointments with us assiduously. She was so apprehensive that, despite the help of 4 liters of nitrous oxide to calm her down, it was a challenge, even for the wonderful Melissa, to provide her care!

Broomy was also a terror at the front desk. She always demanded the final appointment of our day, and--to borrow football great Mike Ditka's description of the late Chicago Bears owner George Halas--when it came to matters of finance, Broomy threw nickels around like they were manhole covers!

My mind drifted to the upcoming confrontation throughout the day, assisted in that direction by my staff asking repeatedly, "So what are YOU going to do?" I decided it was time--actually, past time--for Broomy to shape up or ship out.

If I'd been aware of the situation before reviewing today's schedule, I might have already bid her bon voyage, but mis-communications happen when one works this infrequently, and I tried to convince myself I would successfully treat her, or dismiss her from the practice, and get home a little early, for a change. Either way, I had nothing to lose (unless one considers stomach lining and self-esteem important).

I greeted an already seated Brunnhilde promptly at 4 p.m., with the closest expression my acidic stomach would allow to a smile. (Think rigor mortis.) She nodded a curt greeting redolent with all the compassion of a rattlesnake's hiss. I placed the nitrous--set on overdrive--applied a Dental Patch and topical. As I removed the Patch she grasped my wrist in her claw-like grip and hissed, "Is this shot going to hurt?"

I set the syringe down--fairly calmly, all things considered--and lightly placed my hand on her shoulder. I looked her straight in the eye and softly stated, "Yes, Brunnhilde. The shot will hurt you as much as it does a 3-year-old. And I expect you to behave every bit as well as a 3-year-old would in our office."

Nothing hurts like the truth! Broomy blinked.

After this reality check to the side of her head, she was the perfect patient! When her restoration had been completed, Broomy politely asked if there was any chance her periodontal care could be finished that day, while she was numb. Our dedicated Melissa agreed to stay late and complete her treatment.

There are several things I discovered from this "interesting" experience:

1. It reinforced my strong belief that any meaningful communication should be delivered with some form of physical contact--handshake or light touch--after using the person's name, and always with unfailing, unblinking direct eye con-

tact. All three must be employed if the message is important, and one wishes to maximize its impact.

2. Interpersonal skills are meaningful, but the office is my home--my turf. Behavioral boundaries must exist. Broomy should never have been allowed to take charge. I was determined to:

a) Regain control of the dentist/patient relationship, or

b) Immediately expand Broomy's opportunities to meet other nice dentists.

3. Thanks to my habit of reviewing each record the morning before we begin care, precise computer notes from her last "eventful" visit, and the information gleaned from our morning huddle, I'd been able to carefully plan my firm approach to our interaction. I sure as heck didn't feel in control, but I looked and acted as if I was. Being proactive allowed me to master the situation, as a professional should.

4. After successfully completing Broomy's care I felt great, and my staff gazed at me with a reverence usually reserved for celestial beings...or at least rock stars.

5. Broomy discovered, at around age 65, that she could tolerate routine dental care as well as the average 3-year-old. I believe this will improve the quality of her dental future...perhaps even the quality of her life.

As doctors, and, like it or not, leaders in our community and society, we have an obligation to model appropriate behavior. Sometimes this means facing challenges one would just as soon avoid, but leadership demands courage. When a degree of bravery is required--and believe me, it took some for me to face Broomy--a stouthearted dentist, who can muster the requisite strength, is presented with an opportunity to grow, and thus earn a more joyful and rewarding existence.

Allow me to present another true personal anecdote that, I believe, illustrates an additional facet of behavioral mastery one must attain to claim optimal achievement.

I received a rather frantic phone call from a friend the other day. He had recently experienced some "misunderstanding" with the state board of dental examiners, lost his license for a significant length of time, and was serving several years' probation. I had agreed to act as his state-mandated mentor (although I don't recall the requirement for sending periodic written reports to the board--always a fun task--having been mentioned beforehand). His license was on the line every day, so he was working very hard to get things right.

The "crisis de jure" occurred shortly before he called. He was attempting to place a complex bonded restoration on a maxillary bicuspid for a difficult state-aid patient (for a remuneration of about $50), when he "lost it."

My friend was vague concerning exactly what he meant by the term "lost it," but any dentist who claims he's never had such an episode will probably lie to you about other things as well. I believe "losing it" is like pornography...hard to define with exactness, but we all know when we've experienced it.

That his one full-time staff member was upset with him over this incident, and that the patient under consideration called 30 minutes after leaving his office to request a records transfer, should be facts enough to establish that, however defined, "it" was indeed "lost." My friend's query? "What should I do now?"

My grandfather often advised me that "after you crap in your pants, whatever you do next ain't going to be right." In our scenario, the knickers have already been soiled by the act we've described as "lost it." The time to "do right" had passed. However, there remain ways to achieve superior outcomes, even when beginning with such a pungent mess.

I employ eight staff, have a wife, four kids, a grandson, six cats and three dogs. Problems are not something of which I suffer a shortage. But it is a rare and pleasant moment when I'm asked a question for which I have a ready answer. When I can address a poser with a response that has been fired in the crucible of my dental practice, and proved its efficacy for decades.

I pass my suggestions on, as I know "losing it," in some form, to be a situation eventually faced by all my peers--be they dentists, hygienists, or other team members. Also, in discussing my friend's problem, we will elucidate principles central to success in dentistry and life.

The **first step** was to repair whatever damage had been done to the relationship with his team member (more crucial since she was the ONLY full-time support system within his office, and dentists generally need all possible emotional succor).

That task is accomplished by **ASKING A QUESTION**, such as, "Carol, how do you think I should have handled the situation with Ms. Difficult?" Then comes the hard part: Swallow your defensive explanations--mere attempts to justify your previous unsuccessful actions--and LISTEN CAREFULLY!

If staff trusts you, you'll receive an honest answer. The information offered is not the critical issue, although excellent advice may be forthcoming. More essential is the act of involving one's staff member, and giving staff an opportunity to vent repressed emotions (i.e., "I was so embarrassed by what you said!").

Conscientious listening by the dentist demonstrates that the staff are valuable team members who are appreciated and heard, begins to close wounds, and reunites the team to a common purpose after a trying episode. (Problems not forthrightly dealt with don't disappear, but fester and grow in power beneath the seemingly smooth surface, only to explode--often for no apparent reason--at some later date.)

Dentists generally seem to lack awareness of the important skill of controlling a conversation by asking questions. This querying behavior is vital during new patient examinations. Here the neophyte, in his or her insecurity, tends to prolixity, dissipating this portentous time of relationship-building talking about him- or herself.

We'll deal extensively with new patient examinations in the following segment, but for now, let me suggest that during new patient interviews, the veteran and successful dentist listens, and makes no statement that is not in the form of a question, except to provide information the patient specifically requests. (As the prescient Dr. Omer Reed advised years ago, "If you must speak during an examination, ask a question!")

By **employing skillful inquiry**, the conversation is guided so the dentist can assist the patient in clarifying his or her oral health aspirations. Accurate oral health values and desires must be identified to develop a mutually agreeable treatment plan. Dental care is most rewarding when patient, staff and doctor are all aware of, and enthusiastic about, the proposed final outcome.

This questioning technique is also a critical skill to employ if one wishes to garner optimal results when a staff member has failed to properly perform his or her duty. At day's end, meeting with the staff member in question in the privacy of one's office, a behaviorally adept dentist inquires, "The room wasn't properly set up for our 1 o'clock crown prep appointment. I'm confused. What happened?"

Assuming this team member is fully trained for this procedure, the answer given doesn't matter. In cases such as these--and I've been involved in many--I'll usually nod my head yes as my team member stammers some embarrassed explanation, perhaps dealing with wind directions, or phases of the moon.

The point of my asking the question is to establish that the staff member understands I know he or she didn't get the job done properly, and that this behavior is not acceptable. After the initial question is posed, I say as little as possible, as scolding just makes people mad! By asking a question, one minimizes defensive responses, thus reducing the potential for conflict, while conveying the desired message in a strong, effective manner. But let's return to our original issue of my friend's dilemma.

The **second crucial step** in the debacle currently undergoing scrutiny is having "the stones" to call the patient and apologize. I'd be certain to call within earshot of the involved staff member.

In the scenario under discussion, I'd explain that I was sorry for losing my cool, make my apology, then shut up. (You're not accepting blame, merely expressing the truth...that you wish the incident had never occurred.) Make no effort to explain (justify) your behavior, as such an exegesis might trigger the other party's defensiveness, possibly starting an argument, where one risks "losing it" again.

If one isn't mature or courageous enough to call, at least send the upset patient a letter, and have the afore-addressed staff member type or proof the message, so she's aware of your response. However, I strongly suggest the personal call to be a far more effective strategy.

(I know such forthright behavior isn't easy for the great majority of humankind, who dread rejection, and I don't mean to preach.

But lacking the courage required to do what one knows to be right painfully truncates opportunities to achieve a fulfilling, joyful existence.)

My friend responded that he didn't want to treat this patient again. This is a valid clinical decision. I advised him that, if she suggested returning to his practice (does this seem an unlikely request to you also?), he should inform her he felt it would be in all parties' best interests for her to begin a new dental relationship. Be polite, but firm in this regard, offering the required 30 days emergency care, and promising to transfer her records to the office of her choosing.

Confrontation is unpleasant for most; however, for those who earn their daily bread by serving others, it's unavoidable. Even the most centered and enlightened among us behave in a less than ideal manner once in a while. We are also forced, on occasion, to interface with folks whose two demeanors range from mad to real mad. By managing contention thoughtfully and deliberately, one learns and grows. Two basic choices exist as to how conflict can be handled.

1. To face problems head-on, engaging them in a proactive fashion, as we've discussed. In this manner one can often pick the time, method and turf upon which he or she will act.
2. To passively accept one's lumps, and if you're like me, to ruminate gloomily over one's "failure" for many days.

Dentists are usually busy, often tired, and frequently timid. It's difficult to act in an ideal manner during times of stress, but it's never too late to put a disagreeable episode to rest. Our discussion should illustrate that wisely, skillfully and promptly dealing with unpleasantness is the only viable alternative. Positive action diffuses negative energy, and enhances peace of mind, as when faced, issues can be put behind you. (The alternative for me is to relive the entire affair around

4 a.m. on any number of interminable nights.)

Once painful emotional content has been neutralized by positive action, one can calmly reflect on the incident that occurred, at his or her leisure, and make an effort to define future behavior that will be more consistent with one's values (and less likely to result in having your butt chewed half off).

In our example, where clinical demands, for whatever reason, prove overwhelming, in the future a temporary restoration could be placed, and the patient rescheduled or referred. (As we'll examine more closely later in this segment, action of every ilk should always be explained as to why it is in the best interests of the patient. Here the sedative filling might be described as allowing the tooth to "heal." One might advise that proceeding with future treatment at that moment could result in the patient's suffering a "painful abscess." Information regarding the current state of the dentist's psyche might best be kept to one's self.)

Developing the ability to handle confrontation with courage and sensitivity makes one a more effective, happier person. Repeatedly performing such acts "strengthens" this behavioral "muscle," making future preferred outcomes easier to achieve. Dealing with problems in a positive manner makes one a better dentist, boss, family member and friend...a better person. That seems reward enough to justify the effort.

Allow me to complete this portion of our text with a discussion of how behavioral mastery can be optimally employed to influence others' decisions, thus benefiting one's practice and patients.

High-Touch Skills in a High-Tech World

Modern technology has greatly enriched the dental profession. Yet despite all our contemporary wonders, every tooth I restore resides in the mouth of a sensate human being. (Let me point out, this is definitely not MY IDEA. The majority of my problems are caused by the darn patients. I just can't figure out a way to get paid without treating people!)

As technological advances continue to astound us, it is perspicacious to hark back to the sage advice offered by John Naisbitt in his 1982 landmark best seller, *Megatrends*. Here he wisely counseled "whenever new technology is introduced into society, there must be a counterbalancing human response--that is HIGH TOUCH--or the technology is rejected. **The more high tech, the more high touch**."

Take full advantage of modern computer marvels, intra-oral cameras, lasers, air abrasion, jet ray tooth blasters (still in the design stage) and such. Properly incorporated, these can be great boons to our profession and patients. But never forget that dentistry remains, at heart, a skill or art where one's level of success is determined by his or her dental team's ability to understand and effectively influence others' wants, needs and decisions.

"High Touch" can be literal or figurative, and can assume innumerable shapes. It may be a pat on the shoulder, a firm handshake, or even a hug. It can also take the form of a warm smile, considerately offered beverage, or a simple nodding of one's head to show he or she is listening, understands and cares. The ability to mold human response by myriad forms of "touching" is critical in many facets of our practices. However, if one slashes through the Gordian knot separating excellent from mediocre offices, it becomes apparent that **optimized scheduling control (for dentists and hygienists) is essential to maximizing prosperity**. So let's evaluate how we can use High

Touch skills to influence human response, and thus idealize a key to high production--the ideal daily schedule.

For the most successful of my fellow wet-gloved denizens, a perfectly scheduled day involves one morning and one afternoon patient. Under these ideal conditions, production is maximized, overhead minimized, team stress kept low, and one enjoys performing ideal dental care, while earning a high net profit. Such is the road leading to the lecture circuit! Sounds great. Sign me up!

Knowing this, one problem still exists for the dental team: efficiently and consistently convincing patients that receiving the level of care they require (restoring their mouth to complete health, comfort and beauty), in the manner you know to be best (utilizing comprehensive appointments), represents the ideal solution to their dental wants and needs.

We'll deal with improving case acceptance in the following segment. But imperative to consummating the goal of having patients accept the method of scheduling one's office prefers is developing abilities that permit one always to explain any behavior in a way that clearly demonstrates acting in the suggested manner is in the **patient's best interests**.

Couching one's wishes in such a fashion is not devious--merely the most efficacious way of assisting a patient to make the choice that is optimal for his or her situation. Everyone's favorite radio station is WII-FM...**W**hat's **I**n **I**t **F**or **M**e? Wise staff understand that all suggestions regarding patient behavioral choices must be couched with this WII-FM concept kept always firmly in mind.

Of course, assisting patients to reach decisions ideal for office flow and productivity helps dental teams too. That's excellent, as patients don't understand or much care about what's in our best interests...so we must!

Let's examine some behavioral nuances that facilitate patients' making decisions which we know are in their best interests, but are also ideal for one's office. For example, the **patient's advantages** in completing as much treatment as possible during one long restorative appointment can be explained as reducing the number of times anesthetic is needed (enhanced comfort and safety), interrupting the fewest possible number of patients' busy days (added convenience), and being the fastest way to restore a mouth, thus minimizing the chances of teeth fracturing or abscessing before they can be restored (improving health and function, while minimizing possible pain).

Most dental teams would prefer long restorative appointments be scheduled in the morning. Simply advise patients it is to their advantage to see the team early in the day, when dentist and staff are fresh and performing at peak efficiency. You suggest this because your entire team is committed to being their best during their important treatment.

Let's contemplate additional examples of how to guide patients to select what is best for them (and also ideal for one's office). Parents frequently request their child be seen after school, but it's impossible for our office to treat all the kids who need care after 4 p.m. We handle a request for a late appointment for little Tommy thus: "Dr. Wilde reserves late afternoon appointments for children with special needs. Does Tommy have any disabilities?" Most parents wouldn't take this "special time" now if the care was provided free of charge!

When I sold my practice, our entire accounts receivable total was around $16,000--about a week's production--after 26 years of practice. We'd remained in a comfortable range, from $13,000 to $22,000 in total accounts due, for many years.

Part of this collection efficiency was due to our offering a 5 percent "bookkeeping discount" for payments made before care is delivered. We explained this fee reduction was being offered as "a thank-you to our **financially responsible** patients." Most accepted paying in advance. They appreciated the savings, especially in large cases, and few--even if their awareness remained subconscious--wished to be included among the ranks of the irresponsible.

There are daily situations within the dental office where explanations thoughtfully presented as to why suggested options are in the patient's best interest eliminate conflict, and make one's team look like heroes, who are primarily concerned with the patient's well-being.

For example, we perform endodontics to keep the tooth, while eliminating painful, dangerous infections. A crown fabricated immediately after a root canal is completed minimizes risk of painful toothaches or fractures, while restoring one's tooth to an optimal state of health, comfort and beauty. (Completing endo, build-up and crown preparation in one appointment is also great for office efficiency.) The list of patient benefits derived from ideal dentistry is limited only by one's cogitation, imagination and effort.

You'll need to dedicate a staff meeting or two to this worthy project of finding ideal dialog to persuade patients to make decisions that your team of skilled professionals knows to be in their best interests. Create a list of topics where increasing your team's ability to influence patient decisions would be helpful. (One possible topic could be ways to reduce cancelled and failed appointments. Our "two strikes and you're out" policy has been discussed.)

Role-play common situations, and develop **written scripts** as guidelines. Each staff member should present these ideas in a manner comfortable to them, but all employees should utilize similar approaches that your team agrees are ideal, and with which all are comfortable. (Develop sophisticated **systems**.)

Employing such behavior skill is not deceptive. As dental health care experts, you know what is in the patients' foremost interest...they don't. Part of our unavoidable and undeniable professional obligation is to schedule each offering of care in such a way as to create the ideal situation in which a dental team can consistently deliver exemplary care. One must become skilled in "high touch" communication to do so.

(We all understand that seeing multiple children after 4 p.m., or double-booking one's schedule--as airlines seem to enjoy doing--is absolutely not in the best interests of patient, parent or dental team. However, such scheduling choices might stimulate the practice of the psychiatrist nearest your office.)

Never lose sight of the fact that, blessed as we are with wonderful high-tech innovations, it remains "high touch" skills that assure practice success. Development of these behavioral proficiencies will increase profit and decrease stress by allowing one to work under ideal circumstances, however you've defined such for your unique office.

I believe, most importantly, the ability to effectively control one's environment is an integral portion of having a practice that runs smoothly, and where all involved can experience joy. **For there can be no such thing as success without happiness.**

SEGMENT V

Chapter 11

Optimizing Case Acceptance

Many excellent success stories, detailing numerous career and personal triumphs, exist to demonstrate why any dentist who wishes to develop an optimal practice must remain a perpetual and enthusiastic student of the behavior skills we have just discussed. I can think of no modern service industry where it is possible to excel unless those involved are superb at the subtle art of managing others.

As the last portion of the previous chapter suggested, I believe that, among all the wonderful benefits behavioral mastery can provide to those in our profession, no conduct is more important than gaining patient case acceptance. This statement is almost a truism, as **NOTHING OF IMPORT HAPPENS IN ANY DENTAL PRACTICE UNTIL A PATIENT SAYS "YES"!**

Gaining case acceptance is vital for practices which have yet to achieve their desired level of patient volume. When such offices suffer a scarcity of clients with needed care, the necessity for patients to say "yes" to proposed treatment is acute. But even those practices that have created an expanded hygiene system, and successfully implemented steps to augment patient volume, are like excellent hunters stalking game-rich areas without ammunition, if they aren't proficient in the essential skills of attaining case acceptance. Needed care that isn't accepted does neither patient nor dental practice any good.

The information that follows offers magnificent suggestions for techniques that will improve outcomes for those dentists and teams motivated to provide the optimal level of oral health for each of their patients, and who desire to create a more rewarding practice for themselves.

Merely providing acceptable dental care is not enough today. Modern informed consumers--led by a rapidly cresting tidal wave of aging, and often affluent, baby boomers--demand access to the best available in dentistry, as well as in every other venue. Also, as members of the healing arts, I believe dentists have an ethical and professional obligation--a moral imperative--to perform a complete and thorough examination, then present treatment that is ideal for each unique patient's needs (analogous to the care the dentist would desire for herself or her loved ones), in a **behaviorally correct manner** that allows patients to understand clearly **the benefits of proposed care and the IMPLICATIONS of non-treatment.**

Each member of an outstanding dental team should agree that every patient deserves, at minimum, the opportunity to fully understand how achieving ideal oral health, comfort and beauty can enhance his or her life in numerous ways.

I've worked diligently for 30 years toward this end, and, as I've discussed, attained some modicum of success (these scant achievements admittedly scattered, like rare and precious gems, among a mountainous slag-heap of disappointments). But my ability to attain the above-stated lofty goal has been greatly increased, thanks to input provided by the legendary Dr. Pete Dawson in his excellent How to Put

Your Practice in the Top 10% course, and the marvelous book, *SPIN Selling,* by Neil Rackham which Dr. Dawson and I strongly recommend.

The wisdom I've garnered from these resources has allowed me to increase the effectiveness and personal satisfaction of my critical new-patient examination experience exponentially. (And Dr. Dawson candidly states, "The entire practice is defined by the new-patient examination and treatment plan.") I only wish I had achieved access to this practice-accelerating erudition earlier in my career.

Contrary to most new behaviors--that usually feel awkward, at best--I found the following approach to be intuitively more comfortable, as it allowed me to occupy the role of educator and problem-solver--not salesman--while I engaged in the task of building the positive new-patient relationships that are essential to dental success.

Our New-Patient Experience

We pick up our tale just before I enter my private office to meet the newest member of our patient family. Tonya--director of our new-patient experience--first greeted this patient with a warm smile and firm handshake about 30 minutes ago. She helped her complete a computer-generated medical history, took her on a brief tour of our clinic, then seated her in my office, where the patient's blood pressure was taken and recorded.

A smile evaluation was completed in interview form, Tonya asking questions and recording answers, while the patient studied her smile in our ornate hand-mirror. (No one can perfectly recall his or her precise oral appearance, so a meaningful smile analysis must be done with the patient looking into a mirror. Also, since many questions are engendered while completing this form, doing so in the format of a personal interview is ideal.) These tasks completed, Tonya spent any remaining available time answering questions and discussing our office philosophy. When I arrived, she introduced me and excused herself from my office.

I shook hands, requested the patient call me John, and asked what she preferred to be called. So far, standard operating procedure in our practice...but everything that follows has been improved, thanks to Dr. Dawson and *SPIN Selling.*

SPIN Selling

The basis of *SPIN Selling* is the contention, which we've addressed before under slightly varied circumstances, that **questions are much more powerful than statements**, and allow the individual asking to control the conversation, while retaining patient interest. (Who doesn't love to talk about himself?) Four distinct types of questions have been identified. After I've reviewed the patient's medical history, I begin my inquiries with:

1. SITUATION QUESTIONS. These queries allow one to collect facts, while building relationships. The great majority of dentistry is accepted on trust. As I suggested in this book's introduction, one can't trust what he or she doesn't know; thus virtually all treatment approval is based on mutual understanding and positive relationships.

   Relationship sales are markedly different from small sales, as they entail longer time frames, require follow-up care, dictate an increased level of commitment from all parties, and involve long-term personal consequences. (Compare this definition to the purchase of a book or tie, to understand how small sales vary dramatically from the relationship sales in which dentistry is involved.)

To provide examples of situation questions, I've borrowed most of the following from the best--one of our profession's true creative geniuses--Dr. Pete Dawson himself.

1. *What would you like me to know about you?*
   Thanks for sharing that; now,
2. *What would you like to know about me?*
   (If you have the courage to ask the above-stated dauntingly candid questions, you'll be surprised by what patients ask, and amazed by how quickly such queries help establish a deeper level of intimacy.)
3. *How may I help you?*
4. *What has been the nature of your past dental experiences?*
5. *What made you select our office?*
6. *Are you pleased with the appearance of your teeth?*
7. *Are you planning to keep your teeth all your life?*
8. *What actions do you intend to take to make certain you'll keep your natural teeth throughout your lifetime?*

Of course, these are mere examples. Every question a dentist asks should conform to his or her unique values, and be phrased in a comfortable manner. During these early moments of the interview, it is important to establish the dentist's role of asking questions and seeking information. It is also critical to use questions to direct conversational flow, while building an affinity with this stranger, as one helps clarify her oral health values and goals. We move on to:

2. PROBLEM QUESTIONS. These probing queries are employed in our effort to identify potential patient needs.

1. *What bothers you most about your teeth?*
2. *Do your gums bleed?*

3. *Do you suffer from frequent headaches?*
4. *Are any areas of your mouth sensitive? To what?*
5. *Does food pack between your teeth?*
6. *Do you wish your teeth were whiter?*
7. *Have any problems occurred during the course of your past dental care?*

Identifying specific problems helps clarify patient needs, and begins to increase the perceived value of our service by making patients aware of explicit areas where we can help solve their concerns.

3. IMPLICATION QUESTIONS. Here the genius of the system unfolds, as **consequences of identified problems** are discussed, and the dentist honestly and candidly deals with the **implications of non-treatment**. One skillfully helps patients understand the seriousness of their problems, as they begin to comprehend that possible solutions are worthy of an investment. Dentistry is relatively easy to present, as every identified problem contains implications of a greater dilemma if not treated. (Contrast dental needs with the level of urgency one could generate while selling a yacht.)

As you discuss patient problems that previous questions have identified, Dr. Dawson suggests you couch your query as, "Has anyone ever explained the problems that can result from..."

1. *Bleeding gums.*
2. *Sensitive teeth.*
3. *Joint or facial pain.*
4. *Food traps.*
5. *Missing teeth that aren't replaced.*

6. *Cracked teeth.*

(The manner in which I've presented the question for years, "Do you understand what causes..." risks offending by making the patient feel ignorant. They can't be responsible for the unfortunate fact that no one else has ever taken the time to explain these important issues to them.) Discussing problems and possible future implications answers the patient's implied question, "So what?" by establishing the possible seriousness of an existing condition left untreated.

4. NEED PAYOFF QUESTIONS. After careful discussion, problems that patients might initially have perceived as small are identified as potentially serious (consider bleeding gums and their relationship to heart, vascular and other potentially serious systemic health problems, not to mention tooth loss); thus their urgency is enhanced, and patients' tendency to take action increased.

After patients state specific needs (I want my gums to quit bleeding), dentists can present positive solutions that can solve the **now explicitly identified needs of the patient.** These are presented as **BENEFITS** with statements such as, "If we both do our part we can..."

1. *Stop your gums from bleeding.*
2. *Eliminate mouth sensitivity.*
3. *End TMJ and facial pain...stop your headaches.*
4. *Eliminate food traps.*
5. *Prevent damage that can be caused by unreplaced teeth.*
6. *Prevent pain and tooth loss from cracked teeth.*

After a topic has been discussed, probe for lack of understanding or resistance by asking, "How would you feel about that?" (For example, "If we both do our part, we can stop your gums from bleeding. How would you feel about that?" This information can be even more effective when delivered in an ideal manner, based on which of the four primary behavioral patterns--discussed earlier--this patient fits.)

Need Payoff questions focus the patient on solutions, not problems, thus creating a positive atmosphere. Skillful questioning helps the patient discover--and possibly even inform the dentist of--benefits that would result from proper treatment. (This manner of education where, aided by skillful questions, one self-discovers truths, is referred to as the Socratic method. No learning so influences one's life as self-revealed understanding.)

When every need has been identified and discussed, be certain all key concerns have been thoroughly understood by asking the patient if she has any questions. When all questions are addressed, briefly summarize all benefits of the proposed care, then ask for a definite commitment with a no-pressure statement like, "The most logical next step would be to...." When the previous steps have been skillfully completed, asking for commitment isn't "closing a sale," but rather opening a relationship.

The total fee required to restore optimal oral health is presented ONLY after all needed treatment and its possible implications are fully understood.

The KEY is ASKING QUESTIONS

Lots and lots of questions. Careful probing will help one identify each patient's unique needs, and develop his or her awareness, understanding and appreciation of the benefits your treatment offers. When patient needs become explicit statements of their desires ("I'd do anything to get rid of these headaches," "I'd love to have whiter teeth," "I've got to get my gums healthy again!"), the doctor offers SOLUTIONS TO THE PATIENT'S NOW PRESSING PROBLEMS.

My previous biggest case presentation flaw was jumping too quickly to my beloved solutions "A crown will fix that!" before I'd educated patients to every possible benefit they could receive from restoring their mouth to complete health. This failure to fulfill my total educational commitment often led to partial treatment, or patch-work dentistry.

Also, offering solutions before creating maximum value can lead to objections and price concerns. By increasing worth before offering solutions, one doesn't have to deal with patient objections, but avoids them. Today, I gently defer patients' requests for specific solutions until I possess "all the information I need to determine how to get your mouth healthy and keep it that way for a lifetime."

The information required for any dentist to optimize patient case acceptance has been presented. The challenge now facing readers is one of **entelechy**--turning potential understanding into beneficial action. Few people work as hard to develop a skill as they do to achieve knowledge and understanding. Remember, wisdom exists only when accurate information is **acted upon.**

Begin an action plan by creating written questions consistent with this philosophy, and with which you are comfortable. Don't let uneasiness with something new prevent your growth. Screw your courage to the sticking point, and commit to implementing these ideas during your next 10 new-patient experiences. This is one task you owe to yourself, your staff, your family and the patients who trust and depend on you.

I realize I can't control another's behavior, but presenting care in this manner allows me to enjoy the **satisfaction** of knowing I've skillfully offered my best for every patient, no matter what their final decision might be concerning care.

After this knowledge was implemented in our practice, **large case acceptance greatly increased**, along with productivity and net income. The pace of our office slowed, as we performed more major procedures, thus reducing the frenetic hurrying from patient to patient that had always been our greatest source of stress.

Most importantly to me, **closer relationships to patients** have developed, as dentist, team and patient now share commonly understood goals of helping maintain natural teeth in a state of health, comfort and beauty for a lifetime.

The excellent book, *SPIN Selling*, by Neil Rackham, should be available from any bookstore. For information concerning Dr. Peter Dawson's life-changing seminars, books and other services, call 800-952-2178 or fax 727-821-0482. Dr. Dawson's invaluable services are in such high demand that it would behoove all prescient enough to desire access to his unique expertise to contact his office as soon as possible.

The Patient Wisdom Slip

I believe all will agree that a steady supply of new patients who enthusiastically accept needed care is essential to the prosperity of most dental practices. But even a marvelously thorough and efficient examination technique, such as the brilliant concepts of Dr. Pete Dawson's that we've just considered, is useless if new patients don't keep their scheduled appointments.

How may a skilled dental team maximize the probability that potential patients will be routinely dazzled by an overwhelmingly positive early impression of one's office, thus consistently making and keeping that critical first examination appointment?

As was mentioned when we discussed marketing, a potential

patient's first opinion of one's office takes shape before he or she calls to schedule an examination. In our rural area, this impression is likely to be derived from the combined comments and recommendations of several neighbors or friends, and perhaps completed with a review of our Yellow Pages ad.

For other practices, it might be provided by a web site visit, or after reading a direct marketing piece. Whatever the source of information, something motivated this person to call a specific practice to inquire about, or to request, a new-patient examination.

But once phone contact has been achieved, a new level of awareness, and a relationship based on personal experience, begin to develop. Often the ultimate decision to make (or keep) a complete examination appointment is based primarily upon this brief introductory conversation with a team member. This nascent relationship is the slender strand upon which hangs a significant portion of dental practice success. How can any dentist be certain this crucial impression is always dynamically affirmative, even if the call comes early on a frantic Monday morning? (As they so frequently do.)

Allow me to introduce a simple, brief system that assures the crucial first phone contact always:

1. **Creates an indelibly powerful impression** that establishes your office as committed to the patient's well-being, and constructively begins a journey toward the ultimate goal of his or her obtaining ideal oral health.
2. **Decreases new-patient examination failures**. Initial examinations had, by far, the highest failure rate of any appointed procedure in our office before the following system was adopted. Since we implemented this system, new-patient failures are close to nonexistent.

3. **Allocates exam times perfectly, based on previously identified patient needs**. Obviously Dr. Dawson's level of examination thoroughness requires a significant commitment of time. But how can a staff member determine the exact interval ideally required for any given patient?

   Implementing our system will eliminate dentists' feeling rushed when inadequate time exists to deal with complex treatment options. Also, wasted time when patients present with perfect oral health, and you fill the empty minutes of the examination appointment discussing the weather, will become a thing of the past. (This is important to me, as I hate wasting time...and money.)

4. **Builds tremendous staff confidence,** by creating an easily understood **SYSTEM** (the word "system" just keeps coming up, as I hope you've noted), to guide team members unerringly through this critical first phone contact. A precise, written strategy in place also makes it simple for previously untrained staff members to confidently and thoroughly assimilate this vital behavior.

5. **Affords the dentist significant insights into the patient's oral health values and beliefs** before they ever meet. This knowledge is pivotal to developing the ideal approach to identify, then rapidly and deeply engage the patient's interests, needs and desires during the all-important first minutes of contact with the (still prospective) dentist once the examination has begun.

All these benefits, and more, are bequeathed by the use of our Patient Wisdom Slip. (I'd like to clearly acknowledge that I obtained the basic structure of the following system from some long-forgotten source, and modified it to fulfill our specific office needs over the course of many years. I regret being unable to credit the creator properly, but would like to thank the original author for his or her generous contribution to dentistry, and hope this dialog will further enhance the usefulness of this important concept.)

Patient Wisdom Slip

Date________________

Thank you for choosing Dr. Wilde's office. This is ____________.
How may I help you?

First Name________________ (pronounced)___________________

Last Name______________ (pronounced)____________________

In order to be certain we schedule the ideal amount of reserved time for your first appointment with us, may I ask you a few questions?

Whom may we thank for referring you to our office______________

(Send note and office mug filled with sugarless candy)

How long since your last dental visit?_________________________

What was the nature of that visit?____________________________

What types of past dental treatment have you experienced?

____

Are you pleased with the color and appearance of your teeth?

____

Any current problems?

Toothache ________________________________

Hot/Cold sensitivity________________ Bleeding gums__________

Swelling_______ Lost filling________ Broken tooth__________?

In order to prepare for your first visit and save you time, we would like to send you a welcome package of patient information. May I please have your:

Address______________________________________ZIP_________

Business phone__________ Home Phone______________________

Insurance Company____

It's very important to our dental team that your first visit with Dr. Wilde be a positive experience for you.

Do you have ANY CONCERNS of which we need to be aware?

____

What traits are important to you when choosing a dentist?

____

Your reserved time with Dr. Wilde will be for _____ minutes. You will be able to fully discuss your individual needs and dental concerns at that time. How does that sound?

Together you and Dr. Wilde will decide what x-rays are needed. He might be able to use x-rays from your previous dentist. Would you like us to call and request x-rays be sent to our office?

Dr.________________ Telephone #_________________________

Would morning or afternoon be better for your reserved time? Day of the week?____

Do you have any questions about the practice I can answer for you?____

Is there anything we should know that might make your visit more comfortable?____

If you have any questions before your visit, don't hesitate to call. My name is ______________ and I will contact you the day before your appointment to remind you of your reserved time, unless you wish me to mark you as confirmed today?

We look forward to seeing you on (day)_______ (time)_______

editor's note: A copy of this form used in a magazine article is included with other forms

Take a moment to scan our Patient Wisdom Slip, and achieve

an overview impression, before we begin to study the importance of each item of information that will be harvested during this process.

The date the call was received is important, as I wish to be certain we see all new patients--especially those with complex problems-within an absolute maximum of two weeks of the day they called. We pre-block two 60-minute exam slots per week for those people our form identifies as having pressing dental health concerns of significant complexity.

We record the name of the staff member taking the call so we can assure continuity of contact with this same person, thus increasing relationship strength, throughout the new-patient experience. (Every staff member gives her name when answering any call, as humans prefer talking with a person, not an office...and certainly not those #*#*! automated phone systems that comprise the nightmarish, inverted image of behavioral mastery and are a blemish to the earth's fanny!)

We write first and last names phonetically, as no sound is as sweet as the sound of one's own name...unless it's mispronounced!

The phrase "reserved time" is repeated during the discussion as one of the methods by which we enhance the importance and value of the upcoming appointment, thus reducing new-patient failures. The expression is also employed when we phone-confirm appointments the day before patients are scheduled to arrive.

As mentioned in our earlier marketing discussion, we send a note of thanks for the confidence shown in our office, along with a coffee mug embossed with the office logo, phone number and address, and filled to the brim with sugarless candy, to anyone kind enough to refer someone to our practice. (If one wishes behavior repeated, reward it!) We try to deliver the mug to the referring patient's workplace, where it will be seen-and perhaps discussed- "You got a gift from your dentist? Can I try one of those sugarless candies?"--with fellow employees.

The following three questions (How long since your last dental visit? etc.) begin to elucidate the patient's dental intelligence quota and oral health values. There is probably a significant difference between a patient who last saw a dentist four years ago for an emergency extraction, and one who completed a veneer case before moving to our community. Successful dentists understand that within such knowledge is power!

We'll assist patients in completing a cosmetic evaluation form as part of our comprehensive examination, but we ask about patients' perception of their dental appearance now, to stimulate their thinking about the look of their smile, and to precipitate the process of self-discovering whether they are pleased with the cosmetic image their teeth currently present.

The dentist needs to be aware of any acute symptoms, possibly even see the patient that day for palliative care if he or she is suffering discomfort. Discussing possible (potentially painful) problems also accentuates the importance of keeping the scheduled appointment.

If time before the scheduled exam permits, a welcome package will be mailed to the patient the day the call is received. This includes our office brochure that greets the patient warmly, explains our examination policy and how we deal with insurance, and contains other critical practice information. Before we began taking medical histories on our computer, we included a health history form in the mailing, to allow patients a chance to fill it out at their leisure, and to give them ample opportunity to check with their physician about any medical information about which they were unsure.

The statement "It is very important to our dental team that your first visit with Dr. Wilde be a positive experience" reinforces our concern for their well-being...a central office value. By inquiring if they have any issues of which we need to be aware, we are forewarned of past problems.

Problems as diverse as past insurance mishandling or a previous dentist being unable to achieve complete anesthesia can be addressed in reassuring tones. ("Dr. Wilde is a master at treating patients in complete comfort." Nothing like a little pressure tossed on old Doc's narrow and bony shoulders!) I can also address these key concerns early in my examination appointment, usually to the patient's visible relief.

Asking "What is important to you in a dentist?" affords insight into the patient's core oral health beliefs. Awareness of this primary interest is helpful in constructing my first comments when we meet. Such desires as "gentle, painless, high-quality care, pleasant, doesn't scold" will all be discussed during the course of our complete exam, but it's a **great relationship builder to be able to, unerringly and immediately, address a patient's central concerns**.

After all this data has been gathered, experienced staff possess adequate information to schedule the ideal time required for our new-patient interview. These appointments are generally 10 minutes for kids (we don't complete this form for children), 20 minutes for young adults with no identifiable problems, 40 minutes for adults with no seeming dental needs, and 60 minutes for adults for whom we have identified potentially pressing oral health concerns. These intervals are mere guidelines, and all staff have the authority to adjust them as the situation, and their professional judgement, might dictate.

Waiting for previous x-rays at the patient's request can delay complete diagnosis and the onset of care. It is frustrating to discover, two weeks after the examination occurred, that the "complete current x-rays" the patient was sure the last dentist had taken consist of four-year-old bite-wings. Requesting x-rays be sent to one's office

BEFORE the examination can allow the dentist insight into the patient's current dental condition. (Being able to enquire, "How has the root canal on the upper right molar been feeling?" before looking in the patient's mouth always makes a great impression.) It also eliminates the annoyance of having to wait for past films to complete a treatment plan, or requiring the patient to make an additional trip to one's office when one discovers additional films are required.

The team member closes the conversation by again offering to answer any questions the patient may have. This reinforces our values of compassion and concern, and helps deepen the office-patient affinity. The scheduler also repeats her name, further enhancing the burgeoning relationship. A card with the time and date of the appointment will be included in our welcome package.

Our practice's new-patient examination protocol (briefly reviewed earlier in this chapter) calls for me to first meet this individual after a medical history, office tour, cosmetic evaluation and blood-pressure check have been completed.

At that time, I will enter my private office, smile, greet the patient by (his or her correctly pronounced) name and shake hands warmly. My primary goal is not to destroy the wonderful impression established by all the previously discussed work of my excellent staff. Consistently greeting new patients who have already formed distinctly positive opinions about one's practice and team, while possessing significant insight into their dental concerns, is WISDOM INDEED!

Conclusion

I hope you've enjoyed reading this book, at least as much as I've enjoyed its writing. My original concept was for a concise book of some 100-plus pages, dealing only with hygiene. I knew my personal history with hygiene, and my painstaking analysis of that troubling area in so many practices, had revealed some powerful concepts. And that envisioned book is in here.

But, as I wrote, I couldn't escape the obvious problem that some offices would need more patients to implement expanded hygiene, and achieve their optimal growth. Thus Segment II--most of what I know about techniques to enhance patient volume--seemed vital to include.

As I considered marketing implications, I realized one of the huge keys to my (unlikely) success involved my intense desire and adequate ability to offer patient care as painlessly as possible. Nothing is more important to developing a practice than this. How could I leave this vital information concerning building a practice through comfort out? (To answer my rhetorical question, I couldn't!)

But, even with effective hygiene systems in place, high patient volume achieved, and the essential ability to offer care comfortably attained, success and happiness aren't possible--especially within a service industry--unless one also has the ability to interact with others in an ideal manner under even the most trying of circumstances. I simply had to share a few of my latest thoughts on behavioral mastery with you.

This topic seemed to segue naturally into case acceptance--the key form of behavioral leadership for master dentists, because nothing of significance happens in a dental practice until a patient says "yes" to recommended care, be it periodontal, restorative, etc.

The right staff makes or breaks any service industry, and surrounding oneself with a true team, united by a powerful common vision, is essential if one wishes to enjoy one's practice environment. The finest systems are ineffective if implemented by uninspired individuals. And only when working with others whose core beliefs mirror one's own is joy likely. Though it is not directly relevant to hygiene, I felt the information contained in the appendix on hiring to be foundational to success, and at least as important as any other portion of the book.

The book grew even longer, and more complex, due to my inability to stop offering little nuggets of asides, not directly related to my topic. Many people tell me these seem to be the most honest and inspired portions of my books. I hope you agree. Think of them as the peanuts in a candy bar! In books, as in dental practices, it is often the little extras that make all the difference.

And that's how my "little book" grew; like a camel sneaking into a tent. First the nose, then slowly, the rest of the beast! It took a lot more work and time than I'd planned, but what the hell, I love writing! And I enjoy feeling that I gave every reader more than he or she expected. (At least that's true if one measures a book by its poundage!) Wouldn't your team like every patient to feel they'd gotten more from your care than they paid for?

Let me re-re-emphasize three major recurring themes of the book before I leave your marvelous company.

1. **VALUE CLARIFICATION**. When one has attained absolutely lucid goals, one has the sure direction, and with that the unre-

lenting determination needed to achieve that which really matters to him or her. Precise techniques of goal clarification are codified in *Bringing Your Practice into Focus*. If you need more help in this vital area, buy this book. The cost is about that of a single Panorex film or FMX, and clear goals are integral to sustained, meaningful and fulfilling achievement, not just in dentistry, but in every aspect of life.

(Pursuing clearly defined goals is essential to a joyful, gratifying existence. Moving toward joy is imperative, as I don't believe one can be a good dentist and a miserable person. Life just doesn't work that way. One must become an individual of integrity, accomplishment and merit before sustained dental success--that leads to abundant and lasting joy--is possible. But of what real value is a fine practice to a miserable person anyway?)

How does one tell if he or she lacks clear goals? By the presence of constant and erratic change. If one's values aren't precisely defined, and his or her course thus firmly set, everything new sounds good...at least for a while. Those with garbled values are blown by every wind, trying to develop the practice of each "expert" with whom they interface. But copying another's practice is like wearing someone else's clothes. They might have looked superb on them, but somehow they just don't fit you! Please, take valuable clues from the masters, but in the final analysis, to your own self and deepest beliefs be true.

2. **SYSTEM REFINEMENT**. The journey toward obtaining your dreams involves establishing precise systems, then refining them forever. This is not to be confused with the peripatetic and pointless activity of those who lack precise goals, and whose frantic efforts prove as meaningful as a hamster running a wheel. With system refinement, one's primary direction remains clear

(one is perpetually values-led), but given unceasing thought and effort, I've found one's journey to his or her desires can always be accomplished a little more effectively.

You've seen the impact hygiene has made on my beloved NET PROFIT, yet this is merely one example of possible system refinement. Other areas that intensely impact one's bottom line include scheduling (how to create a scheduling ruler is explained in *Focus*, and this simple technique can enhance the productivity of some offices by 50 percent or more!) and collections.

Consider the varied systems that comprise one's practice, then consciously begin a journey to refine each of them in a deliberate manner, consistent with one's clear values. Steady small steps slowly but surely coalesce to yield amazing final results.

3. **WISDOM OCCURS WHEN ACCURATE INFORMATION IS ACTED UPON**. To the best of my ability and discernment, all the information in this book consists of personally tested and proven ideas. So the requisite accurate information is available. But it will do you no good to memorize this book, if you don't begin to function on your new-found knowledge.

Let me share some words that have profoundly influenced my existence. Author Carlos Castaneda quoted his friend and mentor, the Yaqui Indian brujo (a medicine man, curer or sorcerer) Don Juan, as saying,

"The basic difference between an ordinary man and a warrior is that a warrior takes everything as a challenge, while an ordinary man takes everything as a blessing or a curse."

Resolve to be a warrior, and take all the information imbibed within this book as a challenge to achieve the results you admire in your life.

Every dentist, every practice is unique. I can't advise you where to begin, but commence implementing this knowledge, in whatever area you feel most promising, or most pressing, and thus begin to become the man or woman you dream to be. (Ancient wisdom advised one to strive to become the person he or she pretended to be to others.)

Life is precious, and it is short. Too precious, and too short not to be fully lived. I wish you success in obtaining whatever you are willing to sacrifice enough to become worthy of obtaining, and godspeed.

This conclusion is too precise for me to end on. Please allow me a final aside, one last tasty bonus nugget in this candy bar, before I leave you.

Dentistry is a tough way to make a living, at least for many of us. Some practitioners are too badly damaged to act on this book's sage advice, despite wishing to with all their heart. (I read and studied assiduously throughout my heavy drinking years, and well know the frustration and anger of sensing a dream I simply was not functional or strong enough to pursue.) I'd like to try to help everyone, but especially such crippled souls, by recounting an Indian legend that has had great meaning in my life, and I pray will in yours too. (I have no idea how this American Indian theme materialized. However, I don't believe in coincidences, so pay attention!)

There was once a young brave who was ready to assume the mantle of manhood. In his tribe, this event was occasioned by going into the wilderness alone, entering a sacred smoke-lodge, and waiting for a vision that would provide direction for his life (i.e., Long-term Goal Setting, hardly a new concept).

Our young hero had spent days fasting, praying, and going without sleep. One morning he emerged from his lodge, and saw the golden rising sun, seeming to rest on the top of his desert homeland's highest mountain. Instantly he knew his vision awaited him on that far mountain crest.

Though weak and weary, he climbed. By midday, exhausted but exhilarated, he'd reached the peak, and stood among icy splendor, observing with great joy the spectacle of his entire world spread around him. Suddenly he noticed movement at his feet, and saw a large rattlesnake, made so stiff by the cold it could barely move. The boy leaped away in terror.

"Please," the snake pleaded, "carry me to the desert floor, or I will surely die."

The boy was frightened of the massive, deadly reptile, but the snake insisted he would not harm one who saved his life, and said it was the duty of a true brave to aid the helpless.

The young Indian finally relented, placed the snake in his bag, and carried him to the warm desert floor. There he gently removed the snake from his bag, and set him on warm sand.

The snake struck the boy in the throat.

With the young brave's dying breath he asked, "How could you do this to one who saved you?"

The snake replied, as he slithered away, "You knew who I was when you picked me up."

There is great, life-enhancing wisdom inherent within this ancient tale. I know it's rude, but to reveal this insight, I must ask...do you have any snakes in your bag?

I did, when I drank. And yes, surely I knew what that snake was, when I picked it up. For many years I managed to convince myself that "my snake" was some other, more benign and manageable creature. Not a deadly predator working implacably toward my destruction, but a source of warmth, comfort and fun. It wasn't.

So...any of you got snakes in your bag? You do if you smoke, overeat, have affairs, take drugs, gamble, suffer from uncontrolled spending, eating or emotional disorders. How long will you choose to carry these snakes, and at what cost? If you are reading this, I know you are trying, and thus time remains to put the deadly vices down. You know who and what they are. It is TIME. You too must become a warrior, able to confront and defeat those foes who would steal your life, as surely as the rattlesnake robbed our Indian protagonist of his. It may not seem like it, but each of you has available the power to achieve this worthy accomplishment.

But denial ain't just a river in Egypt. Many, even within our blessed profession, refuse to accept responsibility for their practice or life. These are the "ordinary man to whom life is a blessing or a curse." Instead of the role of warrior--perpetually seeking challenges-they claim the comforting role of helpless victim (thus of a weakling), only reacting to what life brings, blaming others for all their disappointments.

Being a warrior means accepting the fact that you are exactly where you are in life at this moment--be that good or bad--as a result of the choices you've made, and continue to make.

If you don't like the current situation, in any facet of your life, honestly and carefully consider the existing reality. Then, after deep thought, precise goal setting, and the fabrication of written plans, deliberately begin to make new, and more aware and enlightened, choices.

With the right decisions made, and honest effort applied, only time separates you from achieving all your desires. And, trust me, once those energy- and happiness-leaching "snakes" are destroyed, the journey toward your dreams will be filled with a measure of joy that exceeds the ability of the currently afflicted to envision. I do believe it is possible, for all who choose the warrior's path and willingly accept existence's challenges, to achieve life more abundantly.

APPENDIX

Forms and Techniques Employed in Hiring Ideal Team Members

Many appendixes seem comprised of data simply not worthy of inclusion within the book proper. That is decidedly NOT the case concerning the following information, which has tremendous potential to impact positively any dental office striving to become its best. Since hiring doesn't directly influence hygiene, I've chosen to sequester this important knowledge in the appendix, but please understand that the creation of an ideal **employment SYSTEM** is foundational to dental success.

As stated several times within the body of this text, nothing is more essential to achieving practice mastery and professional happiness than working with a team of people who share similar values. Short-term behavior can be modified, but values represent core belief systems, and are permanently changed only under the most unusual circumstances. A strategy based on hiring those with differing values, then working to change them, is fraught with peril…plus just plain dumb.

If one wishes to enjoy a career spent with like-minded individuals, one must clarify his or her personal values, then implement **hiring SYSTEMS that allow one to clearly discern the beliefs of others, and hire those whose values are similar to one's own**. (Recall how our marketing efforts were designed to attract patients whose values reflected one's practice beliefs? The following comment exceeds my area of expertise—nothing real new there—but I'd suggest these concepts are also critical when selecting a spouse!)

So adding people with convictions similar to one's personal core beliefs is essential to maximize proficiency and pleasure within a practice. Being forced to labor with folk whose values differ from yours is like walking all day with a rock in one's shoe. You can do it, but it's damn uncomfortable! Let's discuss a comprehensive system that can help the motivated identify and hire people with similar values, and thus create the cohesive team of your dreams.

The first and most critical step in our hiring process is attracting a large pool of outstanding applicants. In our rural area, I seldom have more than two or three applicants with previous dental office experience or formal training.

To allow the utmost opportunity for identifying the ideal person to join our team, it is essential that we effectively recruit a large number of potential employees who share our values. But many of these fine folks habitually reside outside the group of individuals who customarily consider dental employment. (For example, in the past, two people with teaching degrees have graced our office staff with their presence.) A successful recruiting process must attract the interest of a wide variety of individuals, both from within and without the habitual fold of dentistry.

Our process of attracting new staff focuses around a very precisely worded help-wanted ad, placed in every local paper within a 20-mile radius of our office. We have no dental assistants' school nearby to serve as a possible source of job applicants. If we were fortunate enough to have such a resource available, they would be the first entity I'd contact. (But not the only one, as we desire the widest possible selection of applicants.)

Any effort that will increase the number of qualified potential staff members who apply is a plus. Brainstorm with your team to identify all possible staff sources. There may be opportunities to explore in your location that don't exist in ours.

One often overlooked possibility is hiring people your team already knows. Our team has a standing offer of a $100 bonus if they identify a potential staff person whom we eventually hire. In the spirit of full disclosure, I will state this has only occurred twice in my career, but each time I was grateful for my fellow worker's support.

I personally keep my eyes open with patients, waitresses, bank tellers, or any one else I meet who may possess the qualities we esteem. (If one has carefully clarified values, a like soul is easily and accurately identified.) I have not found an employee by this method, but have identified people who impressed me, and with whom I discussed possible employment, on several occasions.

So cast your net wide, and consider any possible source of staffing. But the reality is, in our rural area, more than 90 percent of the applicant pool our office attracts comes from the following help-wanted ad. That dominant level of response makes the composition and character of your office's ad critical. This advertisement must accurately identify the values you admire as an office, and that you seek in future staff members (only possible when significant valuc clarification has been accomplished). The following advertisement does this job for our practice. Your office ad will vary to reflect your unique values.

DENTAL TEAM: Are you kind, compassionate, people-oriented, and motivated to succeed? We are seeking an exceptional person for our progressive office. We value superior organizational and administrative skills, and focus on warmth, caring, and expert communication with our clients. We emphasize personal development through continuing education, full participation with the other team members, and significant involvement with our clients. Although previous experience in dentistry is not essential, we believe an applicant should be career-minded, personally stable, and health-centered in lifestyle. If you are searching for a meaningful opportunity to grow and fulfill your potential, please send a complete resume to Dr. John A. Wilde, D.D.S., P.C., 1610 Morgan Street, Keokuk, Iowa 52632.

Please place this ad in your paper for one week.
Thank you,
John A. Wilde, D.D.S., P.C.

Yes, this does cost more to run than the inspirational "Wanted, Dental Assistant." Let's consider why I believe the additional investment to be vital to our hiring efforts.

I'd like to point out two salient features of our ad. First, notice the entire description of the person for whom we are searching is based on values, rather than skill or experience. Second, we include none of the normal information usually listed about jobs in our ad. Nothing that says good hours, salary, or benefits. Our position provides all these, but to state these facts about our available job won't appeal to the values held by the people we are trying to identify.

We seek people who are kind and compassionate to others. We want applicants who are already exceptional and want to grow. It's great if they've worked in a dental office previously, but we're not concerned about their experience nearly as much as we are about their innate character. Do they believe in the values that we hold dear, and share with our clients?

We make compromises, of course. Such is the nature of the world! This ad is our best effort to identify the basic values that our team admires. We don't all live up to these values every moment of our lives, but they represent, and clearly define, our goals. (Based on this ad, do you understand why value clarification is so essential before you can begin the hiring process? Without a lucid vision of what one most deeply believes, it is impossible to identify accurately the ideal person you seek! I don't believe it is possible to over-emphasize the import of **VALUE CLARIFICATION** toward achieving success and joy. However…were it possible, I've probably done it!)

For us, values are the hiring process. In other words, in our office, the employee identification system consists of defining the values we desire in a new staff member, and finding someone who lives those values. Once we find the right person, we'll be able to teach specific dental-related tasks we require them to do. But my painful experience indicates it's virtually impossible to change another's values, at least for the long term. (Attempting to modify core beliefs also violates our foundational **Teaching Pigs to Sing** guidelines.)

This ad also keeps some folks away. The people whose only question about an available position is, "How much does it pay?" generally aren't attracted by this ad.

Thus the two goals we wish to achieve through this publication are to:

1. Maximize flow of applications from like-valued people.
2. Minimize the applications from folks, no matter how delightful, who don't share our foundational beliefs, and thus won't succeed as employees in our office.

It won't be effective for you to copy this ad—as your values will differ from ours—but feel free to use it as a template. Meet with your team, and work to create a vivid vision of your future teammate. This exercise helps advance your value-clarification process. Ask, "What qualities do we desire in this new staff member?" Not just what tasks must she perform—although this vital topic must be addressed—but what kind of a person do we seek? The answer to this question defines your ad.

Your ad placed, resumes will come rolling in. Depending on the local economy and time of year, our ad will draw between 30 and 70 applications.

I always review these applications personally, as they are the first gate of entry to our office team. Those dropped at this point are no longer involved in our consideration. Some I can eliminate out of hand. I get rid of the ones written in pencil, or from recent high school graduates, unless they identify something about themselves that really catches my eye. I enjoy the company of young people, and have hired several excellent staff members of the 20-something set, but it is extremely rare to find a 20-year-old who has a clearly thought-out set of values, let alone one whose beliefs mirror our own. (HINT: Our office motto ain't sex, booze and tattoos!)

I am lenient in my judgement at this stage. Again, anyone eliminated now will be dropped from all further consideration, so if I feel there is any chance of a candidate's having the slightest potential, I pass them on in our employment system.

The next step in our hiring process is a **patterned telephone interview**. This is always done by a senior staff member, usually the most experienced in the department (hygiene, chairside, front office) to which we will be adding the new employee. I say "patterned interview," because the same employee asks the same questions to each applicant.

This is a time-consuming task. We have to free the staff person doing the telephone interview from normal office obligations, to allow her whatever time is required to carefully accomplish this important portion of our hiring process. Take a moment and review the form used for this portentous step of our selection process.

TELEPHONE INTERVIEW

Name:____

Address:______________________________________

Phone: Home: _______________Office: _________________

How long have you lived at your current address?_____________

How frequently have you moved during the last five years?______

Do you have reliable transportation available?_____What?_____

What hours are you available to work? ❒ Full-time ❒ Part-time ❒ Evenings ❒ Saturdays

What salary do you expect?____________________________

When would you be available to start working? ______________

Are you currently employed?_____Where? ________________

Can we contact them? __ What is your job title?______________

How long have you worked there? _______________________

Previous job held?________ Reason for leaving? ____________

Have you been absent many days during the past year? _______

Why? _____________________________________

Do you smoke? _____________________________________

Is there a reason you couldn't pass a physical test? __________

Is there someone you consider to be your dentist? ____________

What condition do you consider your teeth and gums to be in? ____

How often do you visit a dentist? _______________________

What was the highest grade you completed in school? __________

Have you had any college or advanced training? _____________

What hobbies or interests do you have? __________________

Are you a member of any civic, professional, or social organization?

____

What are your plans for the next 5 years? _________________

TELEPHONE IMPRESSIONS: ❒ Excellent ❒Good ❒ Fair ❒ Poor

Capacity to communicate: _______________________

Voice: _______________________________________

Clarity of expression: ___________________________

Ease of expression: ____________________________

The staff person conducting the interview must take a few minutes to explain to the applicant the purpose of this call. The tone set with the prospective team member should be friendly and relaxed, even fun.

The questions start with requests for simple information we probably already have available from the applicant's resume. Answering these early factual questions provides an opportunity for the candidate to relax and be at his or her best.

I think the reason for our wanting to acquire most of the factual data listed in the above form is self-evident. It's been my experience that few dental teams ever inquire into applicants' past dental history. As we proceed, you will discover we concentrate much of our attention on the applicant's dental awareness. In my experience, hiring someone who gives no indication of personally valuing good oral health has proven to be an error. No matter how strong an applicant's other features may be, if she has been to the dentist only once in the last five years, and that for treatment of a toothache, she has almost no chance of being invited for a personal interview.

Some may feel this deficiency in dental values can be overcome by proper education, if the candidate has other excellent qualities. This may be true, but it has decidedly NOT been my experience. I believe the questions concerning the applicant's dental history are really inquiries into the individual's personal values concerning her level of commitment to personal well-being. Again, these represent core beliefs, and are rarely modified.

Hobbies are important if one wishes to hire a chairside. Most people with good eye-hand coordination find ways to use this skill. It may be knitting, sewing, or playing the piano, but there is usually some indication of this innate coordination in the applicant's choice of leisure pastime. (Personally, I like to read. If you saw an amalgam I carved, I think you would agree this supports my point that eye-hand coordination will be revealed by choice of activities. At least I turn my own pages.)

I prefer to employ people who are involved socially. They comprise the "people-oriented" kind of staff we are searching for. Leadership in organizations is even more impressive, since it shows the applicant is committed to these activities, and is acknowledged as a leader by peers.

All this information is helpful, but we gather a lot of the same data on the application form we'll discuss next. The critical information gleaned from this exercise is the impression made by the applicant on the interviewing staff person.

If the applicant comes off badly in the staff's appraisal, he or she has little chance of proceeding in the hiring process. If they sound flat, dull, and lifeless on the phone, I certainly don't want them to represent our office!

Thus the most essential section of the telephone interview form—the portion that helps me most in the selection process—is the impression section at the very end. It is here that I ask my staff for the critical intangible: their judgment. The impact made by the applicant on my skilled and trusted staff member during this lengthy conversation is much more important to me than any data recorded.

Candidates who pass the phone interview are invited to our office, and asked to full out our personal record form. The applicant completes it in our reception room, usually during office hours. If at all possible, this is scheduled at a time when the staff person who conducted the phone interview is present. Thus the applicant is greeted by an "old friend."

When applicants present themselves to complete the personal record form, they are again examined by staff. I believe this evaluation to be more meaningful if done by the same individual who recently engaged them in a phone conversation, and thus already possesses some sense of this person's character and beliefs.

This informal assessment (no form is completed, just a brief observation recorded on the top right of the application) consists of such topics as were they pleasant and friendly? Do they have nice smiles? Is their appearance tidy and professional? We don't wish to hire beauty queens, but we do want staff members who represent our values of good health, and display a positive self-image by appearing neat and professional.

(I have a dentist friend who, every time I visit his office, has another 20-year-old, curvaceous, long-haired blonde assistant. I once asked him if he conducted job interviews, or just asks them to send him a snapshot of their hips. I yield to no man in my admiration of curvaceous hips, but such anatomical nonsense plays no part in our staff selection process.)

I can't over-stress the emphasis I place on staff evaluation of candidates. New team members must function smoothly with existing staff, so their impression greatly influences who proceeds in our hiring system.

Also, the formal interview process that I conduct is stressful and takes place in an artificial environment (my private office). So often the true qualities of a person—good or bad—are more accurately revealed during less-formal interactions with my staff. Applicants will ask questions of the staff they would never dream of asking in the interview. Such knowledge, gained through the perception of experienced team members, is priceless in the selection process.

PERSONAL RECORD FORM

Please be as complete as possible. All information given here will be held in *strict confidence.*

Name: ______________________________ Date:________

Address: ______________________________________

Previous Address: ______________________________

Home phone: ________ Social Security Number: ____________

Earnings expected: _____________________________

Work experience: Please begin with your present, or most recent position.

I. Employer: ___________________________________

Address: ___________________________________

Business phone: _________ Employed from ______ to_____

Kind of work: ____________ Your title: ________________

Nature of your work: ____________________________

Skills acquired: ________________________________

Salary or salary range: __________________________

Supervisory responsibility: ________ Immediate superior: ______

What do you most enjoy about your job? _______________

____

What do you least enjoy about your job? _______________

____

Reason for leaving (or desiring a change)? ____________

____

II. Employer: ___________________________________

Address: ___________________________________

Business phone: _________ Employed from ______ to_____

Kind of work: ____________ Your title: ________________

Nature of your work: ____________________________

Skills acquired: ________________________________

Salary or salary range: ______________________

Supervisory responsibility: ________ Immediate superior: ______

What did you most enjoy about your job? ______________

____

What did you least enjoy about your job? ______________

____

Reason for leaving (or desiring a change)? ______________

____

III. Employer: ______________________________

Address: ________________________________

Business phone: ________ Employed from ______ to_____

Kind of work: ____________ Your title: ______________

Nature of your work: __________________________

Skills acquired: ______________________________

Salary or salary range: ________________________

Supervisory responsibility: ________ Immediate superior: ______

What did you most enjoy about your job? ______________

____

What did you least enjoy about your job? ______________

____

Reason for leaving (or desiring a change)? ______________

____

Other positions held:

		Date:	Earnings:	Reasons for leaving:
a. company	a. type of work	a. began	a. start	
b. city	b. name of superior	b. left	b. left	
a. ______	____________	______	_____	____________
b.______	____________	______	_____	____________
a. ______	____________	______	_____	____________
b.______	____________	______	_____	____________

a. ______ ______________ ________ _____ ______________

b. ______ ______________ ________ _____ ______________

Indicate by number any of the above employers you do NOT wish contacted. ____

Activities and Interests

List membership in civic, professional, or social organizations. _____

____

What hobbies interest you? ____________________________________

Why did you apply for this position? ____________________________

In what ways do you feel qualified for this position? ______________

What are your plans for the future? _____________________________

Why do you work? ____

What starting salary would you expect? __________________________

What income would enable you to live as you would like? _________

Please list three references:

Names	Addresses	Phone Numbers
1. ______________	________________________	_____________
2. ______________	________________________	_____________
3. ______________	________________________	_____________

Physical Data

What allergies do you have? __________________________________

What medications do you take? _______________________________

What brand of cigarettes do you smoke? _______ Why? ___________

Would a job that required being on your feet all day be objectionable?

____

Would assisting with a surgical operation bother you? _____________

Would you be willing to have a complete medical and dental examination completed, with a report filed to this office? _________________

What three characteristics best describe you? ____________________

____

What short- and long-term goals do you personally have? __________

____

Education

Indicate highest grade completed

Elementary	6	7	8					
High School	1	2	3	4				
College	1	2	3	4	5	6	7	8

Approximate grade point average: ______________________________

Age completed: ____ Elementary ____ High School

____ College ____ Graduate

Approximate number in high school class ______________________

Approximate class standing ______________________________

Favorite high school subjects ______________________________

Least liked high school subjects ____________________________

Extracurricular activities __________________________________

____

Part-time and summer work ________________________________

____

Class and other offices held ________________________________

____

Major fields ____

Degree (s) and year(s) obtained ____________________________

Extracurricular activities __________________________________

____

How was your education financed? __________________________

Percentage of expenses you earned? ________________________

Part-time and summer work in college? ______________________

Dental History

1. Is there someone you consider as "your dentist?" ____________
2. If you were asked to refer someone to a dentist, whom would you choose? __________ Why? ____________________
3. If you have changed dentists in the last five years, please indicate:

   ❒ Yes ❒ No
4. Do you consider your teeth and oral structure to be in:

   Excellent ______________

   Good ________________

   Fair _________________

   Poor ________________ condition?
5. Were your dental services during the past five years thorough and complete?

   ❒ Yes ❒ No
6. How often have you visited a dentist in the past five years? ______
7. How often did you visit a dentist for preventive examinations?

   Every 3 months ____

   Every 6 months ____

   Every year ______

   Other ________
8. What services were performed on these visits? ______________

   ____
9. Was there any treatment that was suggested, but not performed? __

   ____
10. Was this due to any specific reason? ____________________

    ____
11. My opinion about dentistry is different from other people's because:

    ____

    ____

This is an exact copy of the application we use in our office. I believe (also hope and pray) we are violating none of the numerous, complex and perpetually evolving laws covering fairness and equity in the hiring process here, or in any other section of our employment system. It is our intent to be completely in compliance with all existing statutes. Please feel free to adopt or modify our forms for your use. However, do ask your attorney or someone from your state job service to review the information before you use it, to ensure you haven't inadvertently broken one of the myriad regulations concerning what can and cannot be asked of a potential employee.

Violating fair employment laws can result in severe penalties. Regulations vary with time and geographic location, so be certain that whatever form you use is in **complete compliance with all state and federal mandates concerning hiring**.

The first line of our Personal Record Form states that all information submitted will be held in strict confidence. Be sure all staff respect and understand this commitment. The privacy promised is your ethical responsibility to ensure. As with patient confidentiality, this is not a matter to be taken lightly. Your team must understand no discussion of the information gathered in the hiring process can ever be allowed outside the office.

The first paragraph of the form asks the applicant what level of compensation he or she would expect, were this position obtained. The information gained from this query is somewhat difficult to interpret. I'd never eliminate a candidate based on this response alone, no matter what was said.

If a potential team member lists minimum wage for expected earnings, it could indicate low self-esteem. It could also mean that she really desires the job described in the ad and money is not a primary motivating factor.

If she lists a figure twice the salary you are able to offer, it is possible you won't be able to afford to hire her. However, over the years I've offered a position to people at a much lower figure than what they quoted as "earnings expected," after we came to know each other through the hiring process, and had them accept. This figure may offer some insight into the person applying but use this data carefully, in combination with all other acquired information.

If the salary figure quoted is well in excess of what the position available would pay, but you are impressed with the applicant, I would suggest your staff member inform the applicant of the range of possible salaries when she calls to schedule an interview. If this remuneration is acceptable, schedule the interview. If it clearly isn't, thank the applicant for his or her interest and move on in the hiring process. By discovering you won't be able to meet this person's salary requirements early in the process, you've saved everyone a lot of time and trouble.

In reviewing the "history of work experience" section of our personal record form, I look for a pattern of excessive job mobility. No matter what reasons for switching jobs are given, **a person who has historically moved from job to job probably won't be in your employ long either**.

You'll often find the reason given for multiple past job movement has something to do with "unfair treatment" in previous jobs. At least this is the applicant's perception and/or explanation. My guess is, should you employ them, they will feel unfairly treated in your practice before long. The two exceptions to this negative perception created by job mobility are career advancement opportunities, or a geographic move that necessitated a change in employment. I am even suspicious of these motives. The best employees tend to find the right employment situation and remain in it for considerable lengths of time. I value loyalty in staff. Job stability is one possible indicator of this important trait.

In addition to stability in past employment, I look for patterns of upward mobility within previous jobs, both in salary and responsibility. This information helps me identify those committed to personal growth.

As is the case with my review of the entire form, I analyze this section for completeness of answers and quality of expression. Many job applicants don't bother to fully finish all of our admittedly (and deliberately) long form. If they lack the commitment to fill out an application completely, how well do you believe they will perform if given the job? I also like to study the applicant's use of language. A short form, or one that could be answered with yes or no responses, would greatly reduce my ability to gain insight into the thought processes of an applicant.

When you arrive at the point in your hiring process that involves reference checks, be certain you are cognizant of any employers the applicant has asked you NOT to contact. If the applicant doesn't want a previous employer communicated with, I'd like to know why we shouldn't chat with them, and would listen carefully to the candidate's explanation. Is there a chance that something occurred on that job our potential team member doesn't want us to be aware of?

However, never risk an applicant's current job by contacting an employer without permission. Sometimes the employer is aware of the applicant's plans to leave the workplace, and will be an excellent source of information. But be certain this is the case before contacting them. I would hate to be responsible—legally or morally—for the dismissal of a job applicant due to an unauthorized inquiry from my staff.

Under the "Activities and Interests" section, we again ask what starting salary they would expect if selected for the position. Very often the figure listed here varies from the one recorded on the first page of the application.

You may wish to question this inconsistency. You will see a good number of questions duplicated in the different parts of our hiring process. This is not carelessness or error on our part. I am always amazed at the different answers given to the same question, asked at different times and places in our employment routine. These variations might indicate the applicant has had time to consider the matter more carefully. Other times, it may reveal a tendency to be "creative" with the truth.

As mentioned when discussing the phone interview, hobbies and activities our applicant participates in can provide useful information.

Questions such as, "What are your plans for the future?" and "Why do you work?" help identify values and goals of the applicants, as well as displaying their ability to express themselves.

Under "Physical Data," I wish to identify smokers, a habit I feel is inconsistent with office values. I also wish to be sure all candidates are physically able to perform the job. Many years ago I hired a chairside who couldn't stand to watch us administer local anesthetic. She had a three-day career in our office. (By the end of the third day, she had backed so far from the treatment areas she was almost in the street!) Better for both of us had we identified her distress at any surgical procedure before employing her.

We ask all applicants if they are "willing to have a complete medical and dental exam." We won't require it, but if the answer is "no," I want an explanation. A friend of mine once hired a chairside who had been diagnosed with early multiple sclerosis. It was a sad situation for everyone involved when all realized she wasn't capable of doing the job.

The questions on personal goals and the requested self-description of the applicant offer another chance to examine values and writing ability. As you can see, I like to scatter questions that provide me information concerning the person—not just the factual history—throughout the form. I believe this offers more insight than lumping all similar questions in one area.

Under the "Education" section of the application, I want to see what level of training and/or formal education they have achieved, of course. I enjoy the company of intelligent and well-educated people—hell, I wish I was one—and this information helps me identify them.

I'm also interested in determining work ethic. A detailed account of summer jobs, and methods used in helping pay college expenses, often illustrates the type of commitment to labor similar to my own, and that I admire in a fellow employee.

We have touched on my feeling about the critical importance of dental history as an indicator for potential success in my office. Please forgive my redundancy, but I would give this section of the application most careful evaluation. I have had applicants who were excellent in every area we considered, except their dental values. I have hired them, in spite of this shortcoming, and have been sorry every time. It's hard for a team member to wholeheartedly support our practice's goals of achieving optimal oral health for every patient if they don't personally share this value. I think a lot of you will minimize the importance of this factor as a predictor of employment success (as I did). I'm pretty sure you'll come to regret the decision.

At this point, we have all the factual data we will gather. I review all information obtained during this process—personal application, telephone interview, a staff member's evaluation, our completed record form—and select the people I will interview.

I lean heavily on my staff evaluations, both on the phone interview and their observations of potential team members as applications were being filled out in our reception area. In the past, I have ignored their input, and scheduled an interview with an applicant who "looks good on paper," but whom my staff rated poorly. Usually, I know the person isn't right for the job two minutes after we begin talking. We have wasted not only my time, and the applicant's, but the energy and talent of the team member whose judgment I ignored.

After a thorough review of all data collected, I usually select from six to eight people to interview. I set aside one hour to spend with each candidate. We try to schedule everyone within the time frame of a few days, if possible. I tend to forget some details of our discussion, no matter how carefully I take notes. If too much time passes between the first and last interview, the impressions made by the most recently interviewed applicants are stronger than those made by earlier candidates, so the entire process is biased. Finding ideal fellow workers is too important to allow this to happen.

The choice to do all interviews as closely together as possible often means an entire day (frequently Saturday) will be devoted to the task. Staff members are so critical to the success of any practice that a day devoted to nothing but interviews is a small investment, considering the value to be gained.

I have been forced, by the limited availability of a candidate, to conduct interviews in the evening after work. I think this is unfair, both to the interviewer and to the applicant, because neither party is at their best. I interview at the end of a working day only if no other physical possibility for us to meet exists.

The personal interview is a critical step in the hiring process. Everything possible must be done to maximize its effectiveness. Please remember, dentists aren't trained to interview prospective employees, and most of us are probably only fair (at best) at the subtle art of interviewing. (Truth be told, most of us only aspire to reach the hallowed halls of adequate someday!) Knowing this, we must do everything possible to ensure the best possible chance to gain the most valuable and least biased information possible from the interview process.

Before I greet each applicant, I will have again reviewed all forms they have filled out, and completed what parts of the summary form (contained later in this chapter) I can, based on information gathered prior to the interview. I also create a written list of any special concerns or questions I want to ask a particular candidate. When I am confident my preparation for this interview is complete, I go to our reception room and greet the prospective employee.

I always shake hands and introduce myself to the interviewee. The degree of "cold and clammy" I find in the grip indicates the extent of anxiety that exists. This apprehension is my enemy, as it can hide the best qualities of some excellent individuals.

My concern is not judging adeptness during the interview process, but identifying the candidate's potential as an outstanding team member. I want all applicants to be at their best during this interview. It is a major responsibility of the interviewer to allow whatever time is needed to create an environment where the applicant can relax. A calm, pleasant, informal atmosphere is most conducive to achieving the outcome we desire.

I ask the candidate to be seated in my office. We will not be disturbed for any reason short of fire in the building during this interview. I begin by thanking them for making the effort to apply, and for their interest in our office. I truly am grateful. Often I compliment them on their appearance, and we chat a few minutes on whatever neutral topic seems appropriate, from weather to mutual friends and pursuits. I already know a lot about them from reviewing our forms so finding an interesting subject to begin our discussion is simple.

My staff has checked our computer, and if the applicant has been in our office as a patient, I have their dental records available. It's unfortunate to begin an interview by introducing yourself to an existing patient as though she were a stranger.

Once I sense, by tone and body language, the applicant has relaxed, I begin the formal interview. I start by apologizing. I explain I don't interview often, and due to my deficiencies as an interviewer, I will ask them the same series of "patterned" questions I ask each applicant. I add that I feel asking each person the identical questions allow for a more equitable outcome to the interview process. I also mention I'll take some notes during their responses, and hope they won't be distracted by my scribbling.

I assure the interviewee the questions I will ask have no right or wrong answer, but are simply intended to help me get to know them. I encourage them to ask me questions at any time. We then proceed to the patterned interview.

I tend to talk too much. This is always a mistake, but it is a deadly sin in an interview. The patterned question format limits my tendencies toward prolixity. (My physician brother, Jim, recently informed me that: (1) you never lose weight eating and (2) you never learn anything when talking. Both bits of advice seem accurate, but I have no idea why he happened to share this wealth of the obvious with me!)

I used to spend a lot of time explaining the job details during the interview. That got tedious, even for a "talker." I now hand a Job Benefit Description to the interviewee when they first pose a query concerning working conditions. I give them a minute to peruse this document—which they may keep—then answer any questions they have. Not only does the job description form save time, but in case there exists a misunderstanding concerning benefits at a later date this standard document we reviewed together is available as a reference.

When we complete the hiring process, we require each new staff member to read our office policy manual (a 60-page document), and sign a statement saying she understands its content. This manual contains, in much greater detail, all the information concerning employment conditions and regulations in our office. The brief job description is simply a "shorthand" version, to save our precious interview time.

JOB BENEFIT DESCRIPTION

Three-month period before benefits become effective.
Starting salary $7 to $10 an hour, based on previous experience.

Six paid holidays a year.

One week paid vacation after one year of employment.
Two weeks paid vacation after two years of employment.
Health bonus one-half day paid sick leave per month. (If employees do not use their sick days, they receive this benefit in salary. I want to reward people for working, not for being home sick!)

All uniforms purchased by office.

Workmen's Compensation Insurance.

Continuing education—all expenses and salary paid on normal working days.

All dental work free, except for lab bills. Twenty-five percent off family members' dental care.

Retirement plan.

PATTERNED PERSONAL INTERVIEW

1. What are three things you do to promote your good health? ______
______
2. How do you enhance your dental health? ______
______
3. What quality do you value most in other people? ______
______
4. What kind of persons do you prefer to work with? ______
______
5. What is most important to you in a job? ______
What do you care least about in a job? ______
6. What job do you wish to have in five years? ______
7. How do you react when asked to work overtime? ______
______
8. What additional training do you require to realize your career goals? ______
9. Would you rather be assigned a task and be personally responsible for it, or do you prefer to work with someone else? ______
Why? ______
10. What job situations have you found to be most stressful? ______
______
11. What words do other people use to describe you? ______
______
12. If given a variety of tasks to complete in a given period of time, what approach would you take? ______
______
13. How do you react when treated unfairly in an everyday situation?
______
14. How do you feel about taking on additional responsibility? ______
______

15. What impression do you think you create with other people? ____
____
16. What plans do you have for personal improvement?__________
____
17. Of what three accomplishments are you most proud? _________
____
18. How have past job experiences prepared you for this position? __
____
19. How would you define "success"? ____________________
____
20. If you could structure the perfect job for yourself, what would you do, and why?______________________________
____

I don't believe I've ever asked all the questions on this document of any one applicant. The form functions as a guide to lead the conversation. The point isn't to fill the page, but to determine if the individual I'm currently interviewing will become a member of our team.

As mentioned, I'll have specific questions prepared for this individual, based on concerns raised by the information we've previously gathered. (A common query would be to explain time gaps in their employment history. Often these are occasioned by childbirth or schooling, but you need to be sure you are hiring someone who wants to work.) Usually I will make these queries after the patterned interview is completed, when the maximum understanding between us has been established.

By now you should possess enough information on our hiring system to evaluate the style and purpose of the patterned interview. It is comprised of open-ended questions that encourage the applicant to speak. Each question is couched more to identify values than to establish facts. As this discussion proceeds I evaluate the applicant for an overall impression. Is she poised? How is her grammar? Do you notice a sense of humor? Is this someone with whom you'd enjoy working? Is she able to articulate her thoughts precisely?

The patterned questions begin by requesting relatively easy, factual information, then grow more abstract. You will wish to develop interview questions based on values your team has identified. That is how it should be. My purpose is not to suggest you employ the particular questions of our form, but to establish the benefits of, and provide an example of, one possible patterned interview format.

When the interview ends—usually in about 30 minutes—I ask if our applicant has any questions. After responding to her queries, I thank our candidate again for her time, and promise to inform her as soon as we have reached a hiring decision. I think immediate notification concerning the outcome of the hiring process is the least you owe those interviewed for the time they have invested. This promise of notification also saves team members' time, by preventing each candidate from calling the office and "quizzing" the staff about how close we are to a final decision.

Over the years a number of new patient families have come from the ranks of people we interviewed, but didn't offer a job. Please remember that the hiring process represents your office as much as every other function your team performs. Consistent with our earlier definition, hiring is a form of marketing. (A display of practice values.) These applicants are appraising you and your staff, even as you evaluate them. Even when they are not hired, that judgment will be carried into the community. As always, we wish our office to create a positive impression.

As soon as my office door has closed behind the applicant, I begin to complete our summary form. I allow myself 10 minutes of the allotted hour interview period for this task, and for reviewing information for the next interview.

As mentioned, I have much of the summary form already completed from information gathered before the interview, but I want to record pertinent facts while fresh in my mind, not after six more interviews take place. The information condensed on our summary form will be critical in reaching a final employment decision.

SUMMARY FORM

Name: ______________________________

Application letter: ______________________________

Appearance and voice: ______________________________

Work history (skills and experience): ______________________________

Motivation to work; aims in life; achievement of goals: ______________

Health: ______________ Chronic disease, days missed last year: ____

Education: ______________________________

Dental history: ______________________________

Family background: Marriage, parents and siblings, children, support for working: ______________________________

Social background: activities enjoyed, leadership: ______________

____

Reference check: ______________________________

Comments: ______________________________

____

Job strengths and weaknesses: ______________________________

Recommendations: ______________________________

____

When the interviewing is completed, I sit down with a hot cup of coffee in a quiet place. I review all collected data, and again reduce our list of possible candidates. Usually, by this point in the process, we will have from two to four candidates still under consideration.

Sometimes, one candidate seems clearly superior to all other applicants. If that is so, I will proceed to our final hiring stages with her alone involved. If, during these final steps, a question of her suitability arises, I will go back and review the information on our other finalists.

More frequently, there exist two or three fairly equal applicants. If that is the case, all of them will be involved in the final steps of our hiring system.

The next portion of our selection process is to check references on each remaining candidate. The reference checks are critical. They are also difficult and tricky to do. They are performed by the same senior staff member who did the phone interviews. Often the most revealing information comes from fellow workers at a previous job. We seldom contact the references listed by the candidate, on the theory that anyone can find three people who like them. (Although it would prove a hurdle for me!) We use these sources only if not allowed access to previous places of employment. We try to get three completed reference checks on each applicant still under consideration.

ALWAYS CHECK REFERENCES!! It can save you from embezzlement, drug involvement and many other potential headaches, as well as adding to the information you possess on each applicant. Frequently, a pattern of very strong or very weak references will sway the final hiring decision. After all, these past associates all know this individual much better than we do.

If a reference check is requested by a potential employer concerning a past member of our team, we provide only the dates of employment, and their beginning and ending compensation. That is it! To do more puts one at risk of potential litigation. All my staff is carefully instructed in this regard, because even if the call concerning references on a former employee is received at their home, I am legally responsible for their responses.

If you decide to help a dentist buddy and give out more information concerning a previous employee (as I have done), at least be aware that you are opening yourself to potential legal action.

Good news! Most dentists don't seem to know this, and will often blabber away about a previous employee. One told me he wouldn't touch the b___ with a 10-foot pole. I'd guess he risked his life savings with that comment. Hope he enjoyed it. At any rate, with a little persistence and ingenuity, you can usually obtain this vital reference check information. Just be positive your staff isn't providing others with similar data.

REFERENCE CHECK

"I would appreciate your helping me obtain information on ____________________who is applying for a position with our office. Do you remember her?"

1. When did she work for you? From ________ to ________
2. She lists her salary as ___________. Is this correct? ____
3. What kind of work did she do? ______________________
4. Is she a good worker?____________________________
5. Does she get along well with others?_________________
6. What do you think of her?_________________________
7. What were her strong points?______________________
8. What were her weak points?_______________________
9. Why did she leave?______________________________
10. Did she have any problems that interfered with her work?
    ____
11. Specify: Would you rehire her? If not, why?__________
    ____
12. Is there anything else you would like to tell us about her:
    Comments? ______________________________________
    ____

The key question in any reference check: ***Would you hire her again?*** If they wouldn't, after working with her, do you want to employ her? Review the information obtained from reference checks for inconsistencies with what an applicant has told you. There could exist differences in perceptions concerning some information. There may also be some outright lies discovered. A prevarication on a factual manner, such as salary level or dates of employment, would most likely eliminate that candidate. I can't imagine successfully working with someone I couldn't trust.

The final step in our hiring process is also important. We invite the remaining applicant or applicants to work for one-half day (with pay) in our office, and then to go to a specially scheduled 90-minute lunch, at the office's expense, with all staff members of her future department. You, Doctor, are not invited.

During the half-day spent working in our office, the candidate may discover this isn't the place for her. Much better to find out now than three months later, when you get to practice the hiring process all over again, plus be on the hook for unemployment claims!

Your staff will allow her to complete some simple tasks during this half-day, and see if she performs them well, but the focus of our attention is on attitude and personality. This is not job training, but the last step in candidate evaluation.

The "free lunch" (remember, there is no free lunch…not here or anywhere else) is the last step of the hiring process, but the applicant doesn't know that. The boss isn't there, and often the potential employee will be candid, having a relaxed lunch with "just the girls." Twice I have decided not to hire people based on information obtained by my trained staff during these lunches. (Once I was advised, "You don't need to know why, but DON'T HIRE HER!" I didn't.)

This final staff involvement provides one additional source of information, but its value far exceeds that. If the candidate's future co-workers say "hire her," they have made a pledge to her success. They will work harder to support her, because she is THEIR choice for the position. Such support is vital, if the new member of your team has any hope of being successful. If resented and not helped by existing staff, she will fail. Buying a few lunches, and paying two or three half-day salaries is a small price to pay for this commitment, and the enhanced chance of success that accompanies it.

The next step is for the senior member of the department to call and "hire" her new team member. Our most experienced employee makes the actual job offer, because she made the hiring decision, along with her fellow department staff...remember?

Details of the job are discussed, and a date to begin employment is agreed upon. The department can now finalize plans for training this new teammate. A definite schedule that lists what tasks will be taught, who will teach each skill, and when specific training will occur, will be given to our new staff member the moment she reports for duty.

With our new team member on board, it's time to send the candidates we interviewed but didn't hire "sorry" letters. Before sending these notifications, be sure the person you offered the job has accepted, and is eager to begin.

These letters are often accompanied by flowers and a personal note of thanks to the one or two applicants who came closest to being hired. (Almost always these were the candidates that worked the half-days.) Even with all the care and effort involved in our hiring system, there is no guarantee the person selected will prove successful. You may be offering a position to one of the people you are now rejecting, possibly in the near future, or perhaps in a year or two. You may also be performing a new-patient examination of her soon. In short, you have good reasons to maintain as positive a relationship as possible with the people you interviewed.

REJECTION LETTER

Dear,

I am very sorry to inform you that you were not selected to fill our current staff vacancy. We had a large number of qualified people apply, and only one position to fill. I want to thank you for your time and effort, and wish you the best of luck in finding the job you desire and deserve. I'm certain success and happiness await you. It was a pleasure meeting you.

Sincerely,

John A. Wilde and Staff

Is this hiring process a lot of work? You bet! Can you take a shortcut and pick and choose the steps you like? I guess. It all depends on your values. How important is the best possible staff to you?

Lots of dentists tell me they don't have the available time this involved process demands. Oh, they say they might if they made as much money as I do. But if they continue to hire unsuitable staff members, do you think they will ever achieve financial success? How much joy at work might be forfeit because one will be forced to deal with value conflict frequently? Hiring the right staff is the most crucial part of team building. I firmly believe one can't spend too much time or money on any facet of this team-creating task.

Now that you have all the information necessary to hire an outstanding team, ask yourself these questions:

1. Will this outstanding individual, who so closely mirrors our office values, work for the lowest possible benefit and salary package?
2. Will she accept employment in a run-down, unattractive physical facility?

Consistency and values are again the keys. The staff, the office they work in, the manner in which teammates are treated, and the materials and equipment used, all must reflect one's core beliefs.

You will not retain outstanding people in a mediocre office. Don't waste your time trying to hire the best, unless you are committed to being the finest. Not the Superman of dentists, but a doctor completely committed to being as accomplished as he or she can be. Use this system to find and hire winners, then enjoy the success your efforts have made you worthy of achieving.

Index

R

Share the Wealth with Your Friends and Colleagues

Acknowledgement

A substantial portion of the proceeds from the purchase of each copy of <u>Profitable Dental Hygiene</u> will be contributed to non-profit cancer research.

If you are interested in obtaining more information or would like to directly contribute, please contact: **Scholarships for Life, 525 Lawrence Street, Batesville, AR 72501, 870-698-2355**

Scholarships for Life is a special fund of The Mary Anne Evans & Lynda Cesarski Foundation for Cancer Research which has been registered with thc U.S. Internal Revenue Service and the State of Arkansas as a 501(c)(3) charitable organization.

Share the Wealth with Your Friends and Colleagues

Acknowledgement

A substantial portion of the proceeds from the purchase of each copy of <u>Profitable Dental Hygiene</u> will be contributed to non-profit cancer research.

If you are interested in obtaining more information or would like to directly contribute, please contact: **Scholarships for Life, 525 Lawrence Street, Batesville, AR 72501, 870-698-2355**

Scholarships for Life is a special fund of The Mary Anne Evans & Lynda Cesarski Foundation for Cancer Research which has been registered with the U.S. Internal Revenue Service and the State of Arkansas as a 501(c)(3) charitable organization.

Other Titles by Dr. John Wilde

CHECK YOUR LEADING BOOKSTORE OR ORDER HERE

Yes, I want ___ copies of ***Dentistry's Future*** at $49.90 each, plus $5 shipping per copy (*Illinois residents please add $3.12 sales tax per book*).

Yes, I want ___ copies of ***How to Create the Dental Practice of Your Dreams*** at $49.90 each, plus $5 shipping per copy (*Illinois residents please add $3.12 sales tax per book*).

Yes, I want ___ copies of ***How Dentistry Can Be a Joyous Path to Financial Freedom*** at $49.90 each, plus $5 shipping per copy (*Illinois residents please add $3.12 sales tax per book*).

Yes, I want ___ copies of ***Bringing Your Practice Into Focus*** at $49.90 each, plus $5 shipping per copy (*Illinois residents please add $3.12 sales tax per book*).

Canadian orders must be accompanied by a postal money order in U.S. funds.
Please allow 15 days for delivery.

Order Information

Name ____________________

Organization ____________________

Shipping Address ____________________

City/State/Zip ____________________

Telephone ____________________ Fax ____________________

My enclosed check/money order for $__________ is made payable to:

The Novel Pen
210 Windy Hills • Hamilton, IL 62341

Charge my credit card for $________ : __Visa __MC __Discover __Am Ex
Card #____________________ Exp. Date __________

Place Your Credit Card Order by:
Phone: 217-847-2816 • Fax: 217-847-9922

For questions or additional information, please contact:
The Novel Pen
c/o Dr. John Wilde
210 Windy Hills
Hamilton, IL 62341